Restless Nights

Restless Nights

Understanding Snoring and Sleep Apnea

PERETZ LAVIE

Translated from the Hebrew by Anthony Berris

Yale University Press　　New Haven and London

First published in Hebrew in 2002 by Yedioth Ahronot Books, Chemed Books, Tel Aviv.

Designed by Sonia Shannon
Set in Bulmer type by Integrated Publishing Solutions
Printed in the United States of America by R.R. Donnelley & Sons.

Library of Congress Cataloging-in-Publication Data
Lavie, P. (Peretz), 1949–
[Leylot lelo nachat. English]
Restless nights : Understanding snoring and sleep apnea / Peretz Lavie ; translated from the Hebrew by Anthony Berris.
    p. ;   cm.
"First published in Hebrew in 2002 by Yedioth Ahronot Books, Chemed Books, Tel Aviv"—T.p. verso.
Includes bibliographical references and index.
ISBN 0-300-08544-3 (alk. paper)
1. Sleep apnea syndromes. 2. Snoring.
[DNLM: 1. Sleep Apnea Syndromes.
2. Snoring. WF 143 L411L 2003a]
1. Title.
RC737.5.L3813 2003
616.2—dc21   2003002411

A catalog record for this book is available from the British Library.

The paper in this book meets the guidelines for permanence and durability of the Committee on Production Guidelines for Book Longevity of the Council on Library Resources.

10 9 8 7 6 5 4 3 2 1

For Lloyd R.,
for his faith, support, and friendship

Contents

Preface

One of the questions gnawing at those engaged in sleep medicine, who meet dozens of people suffering from sleep apnea syndrome every week, is, Where have all these people come from, and where have they been hiding all these years? A perusal of the medical literature seemingly shows that sleep apnea syndrome did not exist until the 1970s. Although descriptions of people who suffered from excessive sleepiness had appeared in medical literature earlier, they were viewed as rare cases associated only with extreme obesity. Once the syndrome was first described in medical literature, more than twenty years elapsed before its prevalence was recognized and defined as a public health problem. Today we know that one in every ten men, and one in every twenty-five women, suffers from sleep apnea syndrome; 80 to 90 percent of all the patients who spend nights at sleep laboratories throughout the world are there because they are suffering from sleep apnea.

Although a cursory look at the medical literature would seem to suggest that sleep apnea syndrome is a fairly recent phenomenon, in fact it has a long and fascinating history. In a sense, it had been hiding in plain view, and trying to find an explanation for this curious history is what got me started down this path. How could a syndrome with such obvious symptoms—loud snoring at night and severe, even obsessive, assaults of sleepiness during the day—have eluded the sharp scrutiny of generations of doctors?

I had started researching the subject during a sabbatical I spent at Harvard University in 1984. Even then I discovered the existence of solid evidence that doctors had been familiar with breathing disorders during sleep at least a hundred years before the syndrome was first described in medical literature. But being so engrossed in nineteenth-century medical literature I neglected to devote attention to the more recent history of the syndrome, and especially to the question of who conducted the first laboratory sleep examinations in patients who stopped breathing in their sleep. Aided by friends and colleagues, I successfully located, and even contacted, most of the pioneers in the field, and learned directly from them about the circumstances that led to their novel observations. This gave me much gratification, because mistakes and errors regarding the first people to conduct sleep recordings on Pickwickian patients have passed like a leitmotif through one scientific paper after another over the years. The true pioneers never gained recognition or esteem.

Many people assisted in my investigation into the sequence of events. I am most grateful to Elio Lugaresi, Christian Guilleminault, Meir Kryger, Eliot Phillipson, David Gozal, Terry Young, Colin Sullivan, Chris Roberts, Ron Harper, Bill Orr, Thomas Penzel, Virend Sommer, Mark Mahowald, and Danny Hershkowitz. I would also like to thank the archives of the U.S. National Library of Medicine for allowing me to use some of their pictures, and the U.S. National Sleep Foundation for the results of the Sleep in America survey of 2001.

I am grateful also to the Technion Sleep Laboratory family, headed by Ron Peled, who spent many days and nights investigating sleep disorders in more than fifty thousand people, and taught me so much about sleep apnea syndrome and other sleep disorders. All the illustrating data in this book are from the database of the Technion Sleep Medicine Center.

My thanks to Lena, my wife, who in recent years has been not only my best friend but also my research partner into the fascinating subject of sleep apnea syndrome. From her I learned about the wonders of endothelial cells and the "two-facedness" of free radicals.

1

The Breath of Life

Then the Lord God formed man of the dust of the ground, and breathed

into his nostrils the breath of life; and man became a living soul.

—Genesis 2:7

Why did the author of the Book of Genesis make a point of stating that God brought the first man to life by breathing into his nose? We also breathe through our mouths, after all, and the volume of air inhaled through the mouth would appear to be greater than that inhaled through the nose. Part of the answer is that the ancients believed that breathing through the nose was more vital to existence than breathing through the mouth. "The matter of life depends on the breath of the nose, for hot air is expelled from the heart through the nose, and air enters through it to cool the heart," the twelfth-century scholar Abraham ben Meir Ibn Ezra claimed, and many other biblical commentators agreed.

These writers were greatly influenced by ancient Greek teachings regarding the role of breathing and the significance of the nose. Air's importance to life had been well known since the dawn of history. Hippocrates, the father of Greek medicine, wrote that the body needs three elements: food, drink, and air, with the last being the most important. The ancients were convinced that the reason air entered the lungs through breathing was to cool the heart, which was perceived to be the seat of life, for the heart was the only organ whose function could not be stopped without resulting in the cessation of life. According to the Greeks, the heart was the site of constant combustion, and the heat thereby produced was essential to all the body's organs, as well as to life

1

itself. In the absence of cooling by means of breathing, the heart would be consumed. Galen (129–200 C.E.), who succeeded Hippocrates as "the prince of Greek medicine," wrote in his treatise on the purpose of organs: "I have shown that breathing is vital to the heart of living things, which must be cooled due to the heat of its combustion. Inhaling air cools it by providing the coolness of the air, whereas exhaling cools it by expelling the heat of combustion." According to Galen, breathing through the nose was preferable because it filtered dust particles and other impurities from the air, and even slightly warmed it. (Galen did not elaborate on the contradiction between the air's function in cooling the heart and the necessity of warming the air before it entered the lungs.)

The Greeks maintained that air had two additional functions: to assist in removing waste materials produced in the heart's combustion, and as a necessary ingredient in the creation of "vital spirits." These were formed in the left ventricle of the heart and flowed to all parts of the body, participating in each of its processes. Galen postulated that arteries carried blood to the heart's right ventricle, from which the blood passed to the left ventricle through hypothetical openings in the septum separating the two parts of the heart, and that only a small amount of blood reached the lungs. In the left ventricle, the blood mixed with air to create the "vital spirits."

Although the first person to cut his hand noticed that blood flowed from the wound, Galen's categorical assertion that blood passes from the heart's right ventricle to its left delayed any progress in understanding the circulation of blood for almost fourteen hundred years. In these long centuries of rigid religious conformity, attempts to investigate Galen's claims were perceived as heresy against established teachings and were severely punished by the Catholic Church. And any knowledge of the role of breathing in the existence of life had to wait for the discovery of the circulatory system and the development of chemistry.

The first to challenge Galen's theories was Michael Servetus (Miguel Serveto), a Spanish jurist, theologian, and physician. Servetus rejected the entire Galenic theory regarding perforations in the heart septum. He maintained that blood flowed from the heart to the lungs and then returned from there to the heart. Servetus, however, was also experimenting with unorthodox religious ideas, and he soon fell afoul of both the Catholic Church and John Calvin; he was burned at the stake for heresy in 1553. Progress in gaining any true understanding of the circulatory system was delayed roughly another half century, until William Harvey was finally able to refute the Galenic model.

Harvey, an Englishman, had studied medicine at Padua University in Italy with Hieronymus Fabricius, who investigated the vein valves that regulate the direction of the flow of blood. After his university studies, Harvey returned to England and established a flourishing medical clinic, which did not prevent him from continuing his research into the heart and its functions by means of surgery on a variety of animals. He used mathematical calculations to help him design carefully structured experiments, which proved undeniably that the blood flowing from the heart through arteries was the same blood that flowed back through the veins. Harvey announced his discovery of the circulation of blood in a lecture he gave at a London medical college in 1616. Regarding Galen's imagined openings in the septum and the heart's production of "vital spirits," Harvey declared, "Confound it, I can find no perforations in the septum of the heart, and I can see no way of proving their existence." Harvey's historic book *De Motu Cordis* (On the movement of the heart) was published in 1628, and in it he cited Galen no fewer than twentynine times, along with Aristotle, Hippocrates, and many others, although he was oblivious of the theories of Servetus.

Harvey's book sparked a controversy that lasted for more than a quarter century. Physicians, philosophers, natural science researchers, and all who considered themselves conversant with anatomy and physiology joined the debate. Even the general public rose to denounce the "heretic." Feeling against Harvey ran so high that he lost most of the patients under his care, and there were fears for his personal safety. In spite of the tumult surrounding him, Harvey did not respond to his detractors but patiently waited for the world to recognize the existence of the circulatory system, confident in his belief that the truth would eventually prove him right. And so it did. He was only fifty when his book was published, and he lived to be eighty, by which time he was able to enjoy the sweet taste of victory. René Descartes, the renowned French philosopher, was among the first to support Harvey's arguments regarding blood circulation, and one after another his opponents were compelled to admit that no other alternative was possible.

One link was missing from Harvey's model of the circulatory system—how is the cycle completed? How does blood flow from the arterioles to the smallest veins? Intervention by a microscopist was called for. Marcello Malpighi was born near Bologna, Italy, in 1628, the year Harvey published his book. Malpighi, who studied the lungs of frogs and dogs under a microscope, discovered in them small air saccules that were attached to the small diverticula of the lungs' windpipes. Much to his surprise, he discovered that air in these saccules did not come into contact with the blood. The blood was trapped in minute blood vessels that kept it separate from the air. He named these blood vessels capillaries, since they were as fine as hairs. Malpighi's discovery of these tiny vessels proved the existence of a physical connection between the arterioles and the veins, substantiating Harvey's reasoning and completing his system for the circulation of blood. It was later discovered that the thin walls of the capillaries enable the flow of oxygen and carbon dioxide between the blood and the tissues of the body.

Although Harvey demonstrated that the flow of blood washed the lungs from the heart's right side and returned to its left, thus being transformed from venous to arterial blood, the nature of the blood's transformation and how it occurred were not at all clear to him. Like others of his time, he could only speculate regarding the nature of this transformation. Some believed that the blood fermented in the lungs, consequently becoming lighter and paler, which would account for the change in its color from dark venous to red arterial blood. Others thought that air finds its way into the blood through small perforations in the lungs, subsequently mixing with it and making it lighter. No one, however, succeeded in actually seeing these air openings in the lungs.

The Italian physician Alfonso Giovanni Borelli eloquently expressed the confusion regarding the function of breathing when he wrote, "It is clear from what has been said that the use of breathing is not the cooling of the excessive heat of the heart, nor the ventilation of the vital flame, nor the mixture of the heterogeneous part of the blood . . .

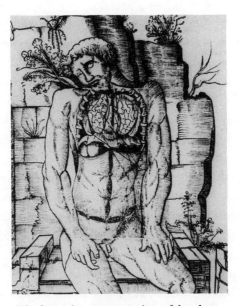

The lungs in a cutaway view of the chest,
a sixteenth-century painting
by Charles Estienne

but so great a machinery of vessels and organs of the lungs must have
been instituted for some grand purpose."

Many more years of original thought and experiments were required before the process of breathing was understood in detail. An important contribution came from four young scientists at Oxford University in England during the course of the seventeenth century. Robert
Boyle, the seventh son and fourteenth child of the Earl of Cork, was born
in 1627. As a scion of a family rich in property, Boyle never had to concern himself with his livelihood, and he dedicated his wealth and talents
to science. Although he is better known for Boyle's law, which maintains
that the pressure of a given quantity of gas varies inversely with its volume, his work on the significance of breathing was a precursor for all
who came after him. Boyle was the first to prove by means of a scientific
experiment, in which he used an air pump that had just been invented,
that air is vital to the existence of life. In his journal he wrote, "To satisfy

ourselves in some measure about the account on which respiration is necessary to the animals that nature hath furnished with lungs, we took . . . a lark . . . which being put in a receiver . . . [and] the vessel being hastily, but carefully closed, the vacuum pump was diligently plied, and the bird for a while appeared lively enough; but upon greater exsuction of the air, and very soon after was taken with as violent and irregular convulsions, as are wont to be observed in poultry, when their heads are wrung off . . . and died."

In a series of experiments using a vacuum pump, Boyle proved that air, and not the actual motion of the thorax when breathing, is the vital element in the process called breathing. Extracting the air from a receptacle containing a scurrying mouse and a burning candle caused the mouse to die and the candle to be extinguished, which demonstrated that both depended on air for their existence.

Robert Hooke, Boyle's assistant and the second member of the Oxonian quartet, was blessed with remarkable technical talent. At the age of twenty-five, he completed his studies at Oxford, where he was renowned for his technical inventions, which included improved air pumps, gauges, microscopes, and even meteorological measuring instruments. Some claim that through his instruments Hooke was the first to hear the sounds of the heart and lungs, preceding the invention of the stethoscope by about 150 years. His technical ingenuity was rewarded when he was appointed curator of the Royal Society of London at twenty-seven. He was charged with conducting scientific experiments before members of the Society, to demonstrate physical, chemical, or physiological principles. The Society, which started in 1645 as a circle of fellows of a "particularly inquisitive and investigative character" who gathered informally to discuss philosophical and scientific matters, was recognized by King Charles II in 1660 and incorporated as the Royal Society of London for the Advancement of Science. The Society provided a valuable forum where persons interested in knowledge of the natural world could present original and innovative ideas, refute existing theories, and conduct scientific experiments in public. Membership fees were one shilling a week, which went toward defraying the cost of the experiments.

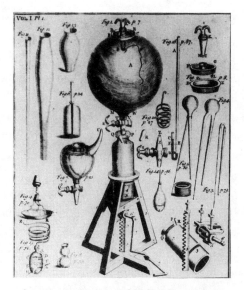

A vacuum pump used by Boyle to prove
that air is essential for life and burning

On October 24, 1667, Hooke impressed members of the Royal
Society with a demonstration of artificial respiration. The experiment,
which was reported in the Society's official publication in just 710
words, complemented Boyle's ideas and expanded on them. Hooke sur-
gically opened a dog's chest and, using two interlinked bellows, succeeded in continuously filling its lungs with air, so that there was no
movement of the thorax or lungs. Small punctures he had made in the
pleura allowed the air to escape, and he succeeded in keeping the dog
alive for a prolonged period. The results of this experiment led Hooke to
the positive deduction that "the bare Motion of the Lungs without fresh
air contributes nothing to the life of the Animal, he being found to sur-
vive as when they were not mov'd as when they were; so it was not the
subsiding or movelessness of the Lungs, that was the immediate cause of
Death, or the stopping of the Circulation of the Blood through the
Lungs, but the want of a sufficient supply of fresh air." Hooke's experiments, however, proved only that the supply of air is vital to life; they did
not solve the mystery surrounding the question of why it was so vital.

What actually takes place in the lungs? How does air flowing to the lungs support the existence of life?

The third of the Oxford researchers, Richard Lower, completed his medical studies at the university in 1665, the year of the Great Plague in London, and a year before the Great Fire of London, which almost destroyed the city. Like all his contemporaries, Lower committed to memory the Galenic doctrine holding that the function of the heart was to create heat, which is carried to all parts of the body through the blood, whereas the function of the lungs was to cool the heart. But Lower did not believe his teachers. In those days it was already known that the color of arterial blood is bright red, whereas venous blood is much darker. The difference in color was ascribed, as mentioned earlier, to a process resembling fermentation or combustion occurring in the heart. Lower regarded the change in the color of blood as essential to understanding the correlation between the heart and the lungs. He observed that the color of a blood clot's exterior pales when exposed to air, and he asked whether this was possibly similar to what happens to blood when it passes through the lungs. Hooke's experiment in artificial respiration provided him with an idea for how to test his hypothesis.

Lower examined the color of blood as it flowed from the lungs to the heart in animals that were kept alive by artificial respiration. He observed that the blood's color was lighter as soon as it left the lungs, even before it reached the heart. Moreover, when he stopped the bellows and the subject of the experiment suffocated due to lack of air, the blood in the lung's veins and in the left side of the heart immediately darkened. This led him to conclude that the change in color must occur in the lungs, and he hypothesized that the reason was exposure of the blood to air. He then went a step further and suggested that the change in color was not the result of the exposure per se but of the blood "receiving" something from the air. He did not, however, expound on the nature of this something. In addition to his physiological research, Lower established a successful clinic in London, and in 1675 he was appointed court physician to King Charles II.

John Mayow was the fourth member of the Oxonian group. His initial training was in the legal profession, until he discovered an interest in medicine. He was a reserved and sensitive man with a poetic inclination, evident in the introduction he wrote to his book on breathing: "The lungs are placed in a recess so sacred and hidden that nature would seem to have specially withdrawn this part both from the eyes and from the intellect; for, beyond the wish, it has not as yet been granted to any one to fit a window to the breast and redeem from darkness the profounder secret of nature. For all parts of the body, the lungs alone, as if shrinking from observation, cease from their movement and collapse at once on the first entrance of light and self-revelation. Hence such an ignorance of respiration and a sort of holy wonder." Some even claim that Mayow's death at the tender age of thirty was the result of a broken heart and disappointment over the failure of his discoveries to achieve recognition and respect from his peers.

Mayow was the first to meticulously describe the function of the intercostal muscles that expand the thorax during inhalation, and he demonstrated that exhalation is nothing but a passive result of those same muscles relaxing. He also "almost" discovered oxygen when he postulated that it was not air in its entirety that was vital to breathing or combustion, but only a part of it. He proved this when he placed a mouse in an airtight container and the mouse died, despite most of the air remaining in the container. He called the vital part of the air "nitro-aerial spirits," but no one gave his theories any further thought and no attempts were made to test them. There are those who ascribe this to Mayow's talents being controversial, which caused him to leave Oxford and his research about ten years after arriving at the university. Others claim that Mayow was simply ahead of his time and his peers were not ready to accept such revolutionary concepts. In any event, it took about a hundred years until this "mysterious thing" in the air was identified and named oxygen.

Between John Mayow and the discovery of oxygen, however, another theory had to be refuted, that of an imaginary substance called phlogiston. This theory was developed by Georg Ernst Stahl, a physician, chemist, and professor of medicine in Halle, Germany. In his book *Opusculum Chymico-Physico-Medicum,* published in Nuremberg in 1715, he claimed that during breathing nothing is added to the blood in the lungs, and that during combustion nothing is absorbed from the air. On the contrary, during breathing, or combustion, something is emitted into the air. Stahl called this something phlogiston and maintained that it existed in all combustible materials. He observed the vapor emitted from the nose and mouth when breathing on a cold day as solid evidence for the existence of phlogiston. Uncovering Stahl's error and removing the phlogiston theory from the study of chemistry required accurate weight measurement of combustible materials and gases. These proved that the weight of material remaining after combustion is not less than the weight of the material before combustion, as claimed by Stahl, but greater. While today we can disdainfully dismiss the phlogiston theory, Stahl's influence on his generation was enormous.

Joseph Priestley, an English clergyman and amateur chemist, was the first to produce oxygen by heating mercuric oxide. Some maintain that his chemical experiments were inspired by a prosperous brewery near his home, which continuously emitted gases into the air. Influenced by Stahl, he named the gas he produced "air without phlogiston." Priestley purported to show that the air he produced was even better for breathing than ordinary air. He tested the new air himself: "My reader will not wonder, that, after having ascertained the superior goodness of dephlogisticated air by mice living in it . . . I should have the curiosity to taste it myself. I have gratified that curiosity, by breathing it, drawing it through a glass-syphon. . . . The feeling of it to my lungs not sensibly different from that of common air; but I fancied that my breast felt particularly light and easy for some time afterwards. Who can tell but that, in time, this pure air may become a fashionable article in luxury. Hitherto, only two mice and myself have had the privilege of breathing it." Alas, Priestly completely failed to recognize the magnitude of his discovery.

It was Antoine Lavoisier, the father of modern chemistry, who administered the coup de grâce to the phlogiston theory. Lavoisier began his career as a lawyer, like Servetus and Mayow, and later abandoned the law in favor of science. At about the same time that Lavoisier was making the decision to concentrate on science, he took a position in a state tax collection company—a job that more than twenty years later sealed his own fate. Apart from his work at the company, Lavoisier dedicated several hours each day to science. His initial occupation was geology, a subject that led to his interest in chemistry, since he used chemical methods to identify rocks and minerals. His studies in chemistry led him to identify oxygen and gain an understanding of its significance to breathing. In 1774, in the same month that he unwittingly discovered oxygen, Joseph Priestley visited Lavoisier at his home and described to him the properties of the new gas he had produced from mercuric oxide. Priestley mistakenly thought he had discovered what is now known as nitric oxide (which has lately been shown to play a central role in neural conduction and relaxation of the blood vessels). Priestley's report on "dephlogisticated air" provided the clue the French chemist needed to explain the findings of his experiments in combustion.

Lavoisier had discovered that when sulfur and phosphorous combust, the weight of the combustion product is greater than the weight of the materials before combustion. He hypothesized that the increase in weight occurred as a result of the materials absorbing something from the air during combustion, but he did not know what this "something" was. Since he knew that only part of the air was utilized during combustion, Lavoisier immediately understood that the gas Priestley had discovered was that same part of the air that is involved in the combustion of sulfur and phosphorous. Lavoisier named this gas oxygen, or "maker of acids," since he erroneously thought that oxygen was involved in the production of all the acids. Thus the phlogiston theory came to an end. During combustion, oxygen attaches to the combusting material; no such thing as phlogiston is emitted into the air. In applying his theory to the respiration process, Lavoisier wrote that the active component of air, which he initially called "vital air," passes from the lungs to the blood, and carbon dioxide is emitted.

But at this point political events intruded on Lavoisier's work in the laboratory. As the French Revolution took its plunge into a reign of terror, Lavoisier's employment at the tax collection company became his downfall when he and several other company employees were arrested. They were sentenced for their part in upholding the royalist past on May 2, 1794, and guillotined five days later in the Place de la Révolution in Paris. "It took but a moment to cut off that head," wrote Joseph-Louis

Lagrange, the renowned French astronomer and mathematician, "but there can be no assurance that we will see such a head in another hundred years."

It was left to those who came after Lavoisier to demonstrate that the oxidation of nutrients occurs not in the lungs but in the body's tissue, and that blood only carries oxygen molecules from the lungs to the tissue and carbon dioxide molecules from the tissue to the lungs, but is not itself involved in the oxidation process.

2

Respiratory Control

Once the role of breathing in sustaining life had been clarified, the next step was to determine the nature of the mechanisms that control it. These mechanisms ensure sufficient absorption of oxygen and efficient emission of carbon dioxide in situations that can be radically diverse, such as vigorous physical activity, while talking, and while sleeping. The early theories attributed respiratory control to the effect of carbon dioxide on either the vagus nerve, one of the brain's nerves that is part of the parasympathetic system, or the entire nervous system. The first to propound the hypothesis that a special nerve center responsible for breathing existed in the brain was the French dermatologist Anne-Charles Lorry, in 1760. He removed the brain hemispheres and cerebellum from a large number of animals and found that breathing did not cease, and from this he concluded that the breathing center had to be found in the upper part of the spinal column, in the area where the brain stem joins it.

Almost fifty years later, in 1808, César Legallois confirmed Lorry's findings by showing that removal of all parts of the brain above the brain stem did not cause any change in breathing. Using the "salami" method of slicing the brain stem itself, Legallois proved that only a small part of it, in the area of the medulla oblongata, the lower part of the brain stem linked to the spinal column, is vital for breathing. These observations were extended in 1842 by Pierre Flourens, who narrowed the area critical for breathing to a spot 2.5 millimeters in diameter on both sides of the centerline of the medulla oblongata. His pinpointing of the respiratory center in the brain stem, and the familiar experience that voluntary cessation of breathing brings about a strong, uncontrollable desire to renew it, led to the conclusion that information on blood gas levels, of both oxygen and carbon dioxide, reaches the respiratory center in some way or other and affects its activity.

Incontrovertible proof that variations in blood gas levels regulate the respiratory center's activity was provided at the end of 1880 by Léon Fredericq, a professor of physiology at Liège University. Fredericq joined the blood vessels supplying the brains of two dogs in such a way that any change in the blood of one animal, following a variation in breathing, immediately affected the brain of the other. In this way he proved that when the breathing of one dog was obstructed, the second animal reacted by immediately increasing the depth and rate of its own breathing. When he caused heightened breathing in one dog, so that the carbon dioxide level in its blood was reduced to half the normal level, the second dog stopped breathing in reaction. Conversely, when one of the animals was ventilated with an oxygen-rich mixture of gases so that its blood oxygen level was above normal, this brought about no change in the second dog's breathing pattern. Hence, Fredericq concluded that the most important factor in the control of breathing is the level of carbon dioxide, rather than oxygen, in the blood. When the carbon dioxide level in the blood reaching the respiratory center rises, the breathing rate is increased, and when its level drops, the breathing rate decreases.

Others reached a similar conclusion. In 1885, Johann Friedrich Miescher-Rusch proved that respiratory control is achieved according to the level of carbon dioxide in the blood, not the oxygen level. He showed that a 1 percent increase in the carbon dioxide concentration in the inhaled air caused an immediate increase in the breathing rate, while decreasing the oxygen concentration by 3 percent caused no change. In the last decade of the nineteenth century, John Scott Haldane showed that a 3 percent increase in the carbon dioxide concentration in the air caused an increase in breathing rate and depth, which was similar in value to the effect of a 14 percent drop in oxygen concentration. Like his predecessors he concluded that the principal regulation of breathing is through a constant follow-up of the carbon dioxide level in the blood by nerve cells working as chemical sensors located in the breathing center in the brain stem.

Only later was it found that variations in the concentration of blood oxygen can also affect breathing activity, and that the nerve sensors for the oxygen level are not in the brain stem but in the arteries themselves, and particularly in the carotid bodies located in the carotid artery in the neck. The first theories about the role of the carotid bodies were published by a number of researchers in the middle of the nineteenth century, but their role did not become completely clear until the beginning of the twentieth century. Major contributions to understanding this role were made by Fernando de Castro of Spain and Corneille Heymans of Belgium. Castro, a gifted anatomist, described with great accuracy the histological structure of the carotid bodies and also propounded the hypothesis that they act as sensors keeping track of changes in blood quality, but he did not say which qualitative changes he meant.

Following him, Heymans proved that the carotid bodies indeed act as sensors, although he made his discovery to a great extent by pure chance. In fact, Heymans was not studying the role of chemical sensors at all. He was interested in the function of blood pressure sensors—the baroreceptors located in the aortic arch in the chest, which also have an effect on breathing activity. In one of his experiments, Heymans detached the neural tract from the carotid bodies on one side of a dog's neck, leaving the one on the other side untouched. When he injected potassium cyanide—a substance that increases the breathing rate—into the carotid artery on the side in which the neural tract was normal, the dog's breathing rate, as expected, increased. But when he injected the potassium cyanide into the carotid artery on the detached side, Heymans found no change in the dog's breathing. These findings were unexpected. If the change in breathing had indeed been caused by the potassium cyanide being carried by the bloodstream to the respiratory center in the brain stem, how was it possible that it had an effect only when the substance was injected into one side of the neck and not the other? After all, both sides carry blood to the brain. The finding was so surprising that, in order to be certain no error had been made in the experiment, Heymans replicated it many times, and on every occasion the results were identical. His conclusion was unavoidable: injecting potassium cyanide caused something to happen in the area of the carotid sinus itself, thus affecting breathing, and not necessarily in the breathing center in the brain stem. In other words, the area of the carotid sinus plays a part in respiratory control. Heymans was awarded the Nobel Prize for medicine in 1938 for these findings on the role of carotid bodies.

The primary result of these discoveries, at least for the understanding of breathing during sleep, was the realization that respiration is controlled sometimes by the brain stem, which is mainly affected by carbon dioxide, and sometimes by the carotid bodies, which are mainly affected by the oxygen saturation level. Knowledge of the conditions under which this shift in respiratory control happens played a central role in the early theories on breathing disorders during sleep.

The respiratory control system must ensure a steady supply of oxygen and the removal of carbon dioxide in a wide range of situations, from vigorous muscular activity, which demands a significant increase in oxygen, through sleep or rest with no muscle activity, in which there is a reduced demand for oxygen. Any cessation of breathing, even for a few minutes, can cause irreversible damage to the body's tissues and even death.

The state of cerebral wakefulness has a decisive effect on respiratory control. Although during wakefulness we do not usually pay much attention to breathing, because we feel that it takes place of its own accord, the breathing mechanisms at this time are, at least partially, under voluntary control. The "voluntary" mechanisms that have developed in the brain's frontal lobe enable us to accelerate or decelerate our breathing, and even to stop it for short periods. But the damage likely to be caused by a cessation of breathing is so great that after only a short time the automatic mechanisms in the brain stem sense the danger and impose their authority on the voluntary mechanisms to renew breathing.

In contrast, respiratory control during sleep is completely automatic, and we are totally dependent on the brain stem's primitive mechanisms, except when we are in a state of dream sleep, as we shall see later.

What happens when the automatic mechanisms do not perform their role correctly? Strange though it may seem, when this happens a person can continue breathing so long as he or she pays attention and thinks about it. People whose brain stem's breathing mechanism is damaged, for example as a result of congenital damage in infants or hemorrhages in the respiratory center area in adults, can breathe only in a state of wakefulness when they command themselves to do so. When asleep they stop breathing, so they must be artificially ventilated. Such a failure of the automatic breathing mechanism, first described in medical literature in the mid-1950s, is known as the Ondine Curse.

The origin of the name is found in the writings of Paracelsus, the fifteenth-century Swiss physician and alchemist, who coined the word "ondine" (from the Latin *unda,* meaning wave) to describe legendary water nymphs who were able to acquire a soul if they married a mortal and had children by him. Legends of such marriages by water nymphs and their betrayal by mortal husbands fired the imaginations of authors and playwrights, inspiring numerous operas and plays. One of these was Jean Giraudoux's *Ondine,* in which the mortal who marries the title character betrays and abandons her. The king of the water nymphs demands the mortal's death, and as husband and wife take their final leave the mortal describes what has befallen him: "Everything my body should do I have to command it to do. I can see only if I tell my eyes to see. . . . I have to command my five senses, thirty muscles, my bones themselves. One moment of inattention and I shall forget to hear, to breathe. They will say he died because breathing bored him."

The division of respiratory control into voluntary and automatic mechanisms, one for wakefulness and the other for sleep, explains the fact that disruptions in breathing are of two types, those that occur during sleep and those that occur during wakefulness, or sometimes both. A change in the manner of breathing is one of the noticeable signs in the transition from wakefulness to sleep. When we want to check whether somebody has fallen asleep, we usually listen to the sound of his or her breathing. The Greek philosopher Aristotle noted that a wakeful person's breathing is fast and vigorous, whereas a sleeping one's is more prolonged and less energetic.

John Cheyne, a physician in Dublin, was among the first to describe a sleep breathing disorder. In 1818 he examined a sixty-year-old patient suffering from heart disease and paralysis who, in his final days, breathed "strangely" while sleeping. The doctor described it thus: "The only peculiarity in the last period of his illness, which lasted eight or nine days, was in the state of his respiration. For several days his breathing was irregular; it would entirely cease for a quarter of a minute, then it would become perceptible, though very low, then by degrees it became heaving and quick, and then it would gradually cease again; this revolution in the state of his breathing occupied about a minute, during which there were about thirty acts of respiration." Cheyne did not attempt to explain this phenomenon, but at the post-mortem examination he found that the patient's heart was enlarged and that there was an invasion of fatty tissue into the cardiac muscle.

In 1854, William Stokes, who also practiced in Dublin, described the case of a similar heart patient. But in addition to his precise description of the patient's strange breathing pattern, Stokes went further and claimed that periodic breathing is a characteristic symptom of heart patients in general. "There is a symptom which appears to belong to a weakened state of the heart, and . . . may be looked for in many cases of the fatty generation [invasion of fatty tissue in the heart]," he wrote. "The symptom in question was observed by Dr. Cheyne, although he did not connect it with the special lesion of the heart. It consists in the occurrence of a series of inspirations, increasing to a maximum, and then declining in force and length, until a state of apparent apnoea is established."

Today, periodic breathing in heart patients is known as Cheyne-Stokes breathing, after these two sharp-eyed Dublin physicians, and it turns out to have particular clinical significance. But in the name of historical justice it should be noted that periodic breathing was first described thirty-seven years before Cheyne wrote about it. John Hunter, an English pioneer of experimental surgery, described the breathing pattern of one of his patients as follows: "The patient's respiration was extraordinary. He ceased to breathe for twenty to thirty seconds and then started breathing again, first faintly, and then with increasing force until the climax, after which his breathing again weakened until it disappeared completely." In light of this, a more appropriate name for periodic breathing in heart patients would be Hunter-Cheyne-Stokes breathing, but in medicine discoverers—like authors—are not always recognized and given the credit they deserve.

Later, numerous clinical observations showed that periodic breathing during sleep, and sometimes during wakefulness, is not only characteristic of heart patients but also occurs following a stroke, in the wake of brain damage, and in patients suffering from encephalitis. Moreover, periodic breathing during sleep does not appear only in illness. Many mountaineers have noted that their breathing became periodic when reaching a mountain summit. There is a story about a famous mountaineer who conquered Mont Blanc in 1875 whose partner tried to ventilate him as he slept after discovering in panic that he was not breathing, and assumed that he was about to die in his sleep. Angelo Mosso, a professor of physiology in Italy who conducted the first controlled physiological experiments on breathing function at the summit of Monte Rosa in the Swiss Alps, reached the conclusion that even a stay of two or three months at the summit did not reduce the tendency toward periodic breathing.

Although there had been some isolated recognition during the late nineteenth century that the breathing of sleeping humans was unsteady and often varied, or even became periodic, as in heart patients, the first systematic observations of sleep breathing patterns in healthy people were conducted in 1925 by Nathaniel Kleitman, the father of modern sleep research.

Kleitman conducted thirty recordings of the breathing during sleep of nine healthy people who, in his words, "could easily have fallen asleep under any circumstances." He reported that the change in the manner of breathing at the falling asleep stage was surprising. In half of the experiments, immediately after the subjects fell asleep their breathing became irregular, in some cases in a pattern that appeared astonishingly similar to the Cheyne-Stokes breathing of heart patients. The periodic pattern then disappeared, and breathing returned to its normal pattern only when the subject sank into deep sleep, or awakened.

Some forty years later, two Swedish researchers, Knut Bulow and David H. Ingvar, conducted a similar study, but with modern measuring methods. Unlike Kleitman, who observed his subjects in order to determine whether they were asleep or awake, Bulow and Ingvar recorded the subjects' brain waves to track the course of falling asleep. They found that each variation in brain waves marked a transition from wakefulness to sleep, and was linked to breathing irregularity, just as Kleitman had reported. Bulow and Ingvar explained this breathing instability by suggesting that there is a reduction in sensitivity of the brain stem respiratory center to carbon dioxide during the process of falling asleep. This caused breathing irregularity in the form of fluctuation between shallow, inefficient breathing—resulting from an insufficient reaction to carbon dioxide levels—and deep, rapid breathing that compensated for it. Deep breathing causes a drop in the carbon dioxide level in the blood, and occurs as a consequence of a slowing down of breathing or even a brief cessation of it, and so on.

On the basis of their observations, Bulow and Ingvar reached two important conclusions. First, because of the proximity of the respiratory centers to the sleep control centers in the brain stem, there is a mutual effect between the level of wakefulness and breathing functionality. Second, because of this link, it may be expected that patients who are experiencing disorders in their wakefulness levels will also suffer from breathing disorders when they fall asleep. As we shall see, their hypothesis was absolutely correct.

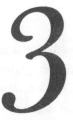

The First Pickwickian

It is easy to understand why the periodic breathing of heart patients caught the eye of Hunter, Cheyne, and Stokes even two hundred years ago. Heart patients, especially in the terminal stages of their illness, are under the close supervision of either their family or their doctors. People close to heart patients while they are asleep cannot avoid noticing their strange breathing. The patient's chest pumps like a bellows for about half a minute, and then, very slowly, its activity wanes or stops completely for a similar period, over and over again. Sleep apnea syndrome, which is likewise characterized by a nightly struggle for each and every breath, did not appear in medical literature until the second half of the twentieth century, some 150 years after the first description of Cheyne-Stokes breathing. Why a description of the syndrome was so long in coming is a question that has occupied me ever since I first witnessed the nocturnal drama of sleep apnea patients. I found it strange that a syndrome whose symptoms are so clear—loud snoring that can be heard from a distance, restless sleep interrupted by intermittent cessation of breathing sometimes lasting for a minute or more, and acute sleepiness that makes daytime functioning difficult—remained hidden from the eyes of many generations of physicians.

In 1984 I was on sabbatical at Harvard University's medical school in Boston. In this relaxed atmosphere, without any formal, everyday ac-

ademic obligations, I became interested in making a historical study of
sleep disorders. Ever since I was in high school, where I had enjoyed history but later gravitated toward the natural sciences, I have been fascinated
by the historical aspect of scientific discoveries. Harvard was the ideal
place to study the history of medicine. The basement of the Conway Library at the Harvard School of Medicine is a treasure trove of medical history, but even more important, on the library's top floor, in a special section where rare books and papers are kept, I found a team of librarians
who welcomed me with extraordinary enthusiasm. It appeared that the
few visitors who took the trouble to burrow through the stacks of disinte-
grating medical journals and yellowing books immediately became hon-
ored guests who were pampered by the entire team. Two years later, when
I saw *The Name of the Rose,* in which Sean Connery's character unearthed
the secrets of a monks' library that jealously preserved ancient Greek
writings, it reminded me of the rare book section of the Conway Library.

The library revealed to what extent modern sleep researchers were
unaware of the medical literature on sleep disorders from before the era
of sleep laboratory research. Sleep disorders, it turned out, had not only
attracted the inquiring eyes of nineteenth-century physicians, but they
had merited detailed, even juicy descriptions. In a catalog of nineteenth-
century medical papers, under the entries for "Sleep" and "Sleep disorders," I discovered more than 900 medical articles. Of these, 316 dealt
with various forms of "Excessive sleepiness." These papers opened the
road to further elucidation of the history of sleep disordered breathing.

Falling Asleep Holding a Duck

Breathing disorders in sleep, including the one known today as sleep
apnea syndrome, were described in great detail in the nineteenth century, as long as 150 years ago. In 1877, for example, W. H. Broadbent, a
doctor from St. Mary's Hospital in London, published an article in *The
Lancet* on Cheyne-Stokes breathing. At the conclusion of the article, he
described a strange case of sleep disordered breathing that was only
"similar to Cheyne-Stokes breathing":

When a person, especially advanced in years, is lying on his back in heavy sleep and snoring loudly, it very commonly happens that every now and then the inspiration fails to over-come the resistance in the pharynx of which stretor or snoring is the audible sign, and there will be perfect silence through two, three, or four respiratory periods, in which there are in-effectual chest movements; finally, air enters with a loud snort, after which there are several compensatory deep inspirations before the breathing settles down to its usual rhythm. In the case to which I allude there was something more than this. The snoring ceased at regular intervals, and the pause was so long as to excite attention, and indeed alarm.

Broadbent was aware that suspensions of breathing, or apneas, occurred only in sleep and worsened when the patient lay on his or her back, and he complained that his contemporaries tended to ignore this fact. He ended his article by declaring, "All the theories that have attempted to explain this phenomenon are inadequate and I have none of my own."

Eleven years later two further articles were published that were no less detailed or descriptive. On February 8, 1888, Richard Caton of Liverpool, who gained his place in medical history as the discoverer of the brain's electrical activity, presented a most interesting case to the Clinical Society of London, a case he erroneously described as one of narcolepsy.

The patient, a thirty-seven-year-old poulterer, complained of great sleepiness that appeared at the same time as a marked increase in his weight. His condition was extremely severe: "The moment he sat down in his chair sleep came on, and even when standing or walking he would sink into sleep. Constantly while serving customers in his shop, sleep would come on as he stood by the counter, he would wake and find himself holding in his hand the duck or chicken which he had been selling to a customer a quarter of an hour before, the customer having in the meantime departed." A description of the unfortunate poulterer's sleep leaves no doubt regarding the nature of the disorder from which he suffered:

When in sound sleep a very peculiar state of the glottis is observed, a spasmodic closure entirely suspending respiration. The thorax and abdomen are seen to heave from fruitless contractions of the inspiratory and expiratory muscles; their efforts increase in violence for about a minute or a minute and a half, the skin meantime becoming more and more cyanosed, until at last, when the condition to the onlooker is most alarming, the glottic obstruction yields, a series of long inspirations and expirations follows, and cyanosis disappears. This acute dyspnoeic attack does not awaken the patient. . . . If in the midst of the dyspnoeic attack he is forcibly aroused, the glottic spasm at once relaxes. The night nurses state that these attacks go on throughout the night.

Loyal to the theory popular at the time that the source of sleep is in toxins that affect the nervous system, Caton assumed that the case he described was the result of a toxin that acted only on the glottal muscles, although he admitted that he had no idea why this should be so. Following intensive treatment with a number of drugs, the sleepiness passed, and to the patient's joy he was able to read a newspaper "for half an hour, every now and then, without falling asleep." Significantly, the patient also lost weight at the same time as an improvement occurred both in his sleep and in his level of wakefulness.

The second case is almost identical to the first, and was reported by Alexander Morrison, also an Englishman. The case was that of a very obese sixty-three-year-old man who had suffered for fifteen years from sleepiness, which became progressively more acute as the years went by: "He would fall asleep while playing a game of cards, the cards suddenly dropping out of his hand on the table, and he beginning to snore, and his face becoming darkly engorged until his companions succeeded in arousing him. . . . I have myself observed him asleep in bed with an intensely cyanotic countenance, a condition from which he was roused after a snorting and choking sound had issued from his respiratory passages, the cyanosis then gradually disappeared."

Morrison was aware of Caton's description and even compared the two cases, but he quite rightly disagreed that this was a case of narcolepsy. Although there is no doubt that Broadbent, Caton, and Morrison described with great accuracy the sleep of people suffering from sleep apnea, and further described serious disorders in their wakefulness during the day, not one of them claimed that the problem was a disorder unique to sleep.

The American physician Silas Weir Mitchell was among the first to suggest that there are breathing disorders that "occur solely during sleep." Mitchell, who had also made a name for himself as the author of novellas and poems, was one of the first neurologists and toxicologists in the United States, and among his other interests was sleep and its disorders. In his article "On Sleep Disorders," published in 1850, Mitchell defined "Breathing failure in sleep" as follows: "Where, for some reason, the respiratory centers are diseased or disordered, a man may possess enough ganglionic energy to carry on breathing well while the will can supplement the automatic activity of the lower centers. But in sleep, these being not quite competent, and the volition off guard, there ensues a gradual failure of respiration, and the man awakes with a sense of impending suffocation. This is not to be confounded with the hysterical sleep symptom of sense of suffocation, which is probably closer to the phenomenon of nightmares, and is followed by or associated with fear, and is soon lost on awakening."

Mitchell's experience in sleep breathing disorders totaled four cases, one of which he described in detail: "Mr. C., aged fifty-six years, had posterior sclerosis, but gave no evidence in the day of respiratory incompetence, although he was distinctly far in the paralytic state. When in deep sleep he began to breathe less and less deeply, and at last, for a few seconds, not to breathe at all. At this moment, he moved, twitched, and at last awakened with evidences of commencing apnea in the color of the lips, tongue, and nails. . . . As the time went on the trouble increased, and whenever he fell asleep respiration ceased abruptly. He was finally worn out with loss of sleep and died suddenly in one of these onsets of respiratory failure." From this description it seems safe to conclude that the patient had been enduring the Ondine Curse: at the end of his life, his automatic breathing centers were not working at all during sleep.

Joe: The First Pickwickian

Richard Caton's picturesque description of the patient who stopped breathing while asleep, delivered before the Clinical Society of London, is a benchmark in the history of sleep apnea syndrome, but not only because of the actual description of the case. Christopher Heath, who was president of the Clinical Society and chaired the discussion following Caton's presentation, was the first to point out the great similarity between obese, sleepy patients and the fat boy Joe from *The Pickwick Papers,* by Charles Dickens, first published in 1835. In chapters 53 and 54 we encounter Joe under very embarrassing circumstances:

> A most violent and startling knocking was heard at the door; it was not an ordinary double knock, but a constant and uninterrupted succession of the loudest single raps, as if the knocker were endowed with the perpetual motion, or the person outside had forgotten to leave off.
>
> "Dear me, what's that!" exclaimed Parker, starting.
>
> "I think it is a knock at the door," said Mr. Pickwick, as if there could be the smallest doubt of the fact! . . .
>
> . . . "I'll answer the door in one moment, sir," replied the clerk.
>
> The knocker appeared to hear the response, and to assert that it was quite impossible he could wait so long. It made a stupendous uproar.
>
> Mr. Lowten . . . hurried to the door, and turned the handle . . .
>
> The object that presented itself to the eyes of the astonished clerk, was a boy—a wonderfully fat boy—habited as a serving lad, standing upright on the mat, with his eyes closed as if in sleep. He had never seen such a fat boy . . .
>
> "What's the matter?" inquired the clerk.
>
> The extraordinary boy replied not a word; but he nodded once, and seemed, to the clerk's imagination, to snore feebly.
>
> "Where do you come from?" inquired the clerk.

The boy made no sign. He breathed heavily, but in all other respects was motionless.

The clerk repeated the question thrice, and receiving no answer, prepared to shut the door, when the boy suddenly opened his eyes, winked several times, sneezed once, and raised his hand as if to repeat the knocking. Finding the door open, he stared about him with astonishment, and at length fixed his eyes on Mr. Lowten's face.

"What the devil do you knock in that way for?" inquired the clerk, angrily.

"Which way?" said the boy, in a slow and sleepy voice.

"Why, like forty hackney-coachmen," replied the clerk.

"Because master said, I wasn't to leave off knocking till they opened the door, for fear I should go to sleep," said the boy.

Dickens, who based his characters on real people from his surroundings, got the inspiration for Joe from the fat, sleepy son of the publican whose inn he occasionally visited. His fictional character resonated with people, and the association stuck. The renowned Oxford professor of medicine Sir William Osler, in the eighth edition of his celebrated textbook *Principles and Practice of Medicine* (first published in 1892), joined a number of others in suggesting the term "Pickwickian" to describe obese and sleepy patients. A hundred years after Dickens created the character, "Pickwickian syndrome" was an established medical coinage for the combination of obesity and extreme sleepiness.

Another late-nineteenth-century physician also noted the similarity between Dickens's Joe and an obese, sleepy youth who was in his care, and in the course of his description he mentioned an issue that persists as a major concern today. The doctor, Byron Bramwell, wrote: "This boy—presented in a minor degree a condition similar to the fat boy in *Pickwick Papers*—whenever he sits down he seems to go to sleep. He is a post boy by occupation and while driving he often goes to sleep on his box." Drivers falling asleep at the reins—or at the wheel—and causing an accident are a serious medical and public problem to this day, particularly regarding the matter of liability. The cumulative economic damage from acci-

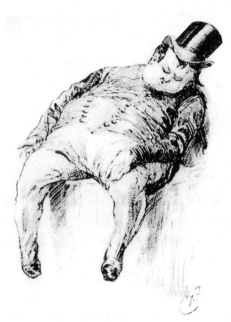

Joe, the Pickwickian boy, from the second
edition of Charles Dickens,
The Pickwick Papers

dents caused by drivers falling asleep is estimated at the astronomical figure of $120 *billion* annually. In the United States alone, estimates are that
thousands of fatalities each year result from drivers falling asleep and causing accidents. Yet insurance companies apparently remain unaware that
many professional drivers are prone to accidents because of daytime sleepiness, which in turn is the consequence of sleep disordered breathing.

"Shut Your Mouth and Save Your Life"

At this point it is important to mention the contribution of George
Catlin, the nineteenth-century American lawyer, artist, and amateur an-
thropologist. Catlin also devoted an entire book to the merits of breathing through the nose while asleep, and the dire perils of sleeping while
breathing through the mouth, thereby putting himself ahead of his time
by many years. Americans mostly know Catlin as a painter of American

Indians, and his works, which depict life on the Great Plains before the white man's drive westward, are displayed at the Smithsonian Institution in Washington, D.C. But Catlin also occupies a place of honor in the history of sleep breathing disorders, and this contribution, too, is linked to his adventures in the Wild West.

Catlin was born in 1796 in the tiny, fifty-house Pennsylvania village of Wilkes-Barre. When he was four his family moved to a farm in New York State, where his great love of nature and painting was born. Although he studied law and even practiced it for about two years, the painting bug gave him no rest. In 1823 he left to settle in Philadelphia, where he opened a studio and painted portraits and miniatures. The idea of documenting the life and customs of Native Americans came to him when an Indian delegation passed through Philadelphia on its way to Washington. He was so impressed by their dress and colorful ceremonial appearance that he decided to paint them. He embarked on his first journey westward in 1830, and this, like all journeys westward at the time, began in St. Louis.

The voyage aboard the steamer *Yellowstone* took him two thousand miles up the Missouri River to the small trading post of Porte Pierre, which today is in South Dakota. From there he began wandering among the native tribes, quickly making a name for himself as a "medicine painter," an artist with magical and medicinal attributes. Catlin, who learned how to communicate in the natives' languages, meticulously documented their lifestyle, painting men, women, and children engaged in their rituals, hunting, and everyday activities. He returned home after two years, and only a few months later joined an army research party that was going to the Southwest, the territory of the Comanches, who were known as fierce warriors. Although forced to return early from this expedition because of illness, Catlin managed to capture the Comanche braves and their lifestyle on canvas. His third expedition to the West was to Minnesota, where he traveled the regions noted for their red clay, from which the Indians of all tribes fashioned their peace pipes. The area was considered sacred, and Catlin was among the first white men permitted to visit it, even collecting samples of the red clay that to this day bears his name, catlinite. In 1841 he published his experiences in the American wilderness in his two-volume book, *Manners, Customs, and Conditions of the North American Indians,* with some two hundred of his own illustrations.

Catlin viewed himself more as an ethnographer than as a painter and saw his primary mission as documenting the life and customs of the Native Americans. One of his books was devoted to a discussion of why the "Redskins" were healthier than the "Palefaces." This book, which meanwhile has been almost completely forgotten, was first published in 1861 and gained great popularity, with five reprints following the first edition. Catlin titled the book *The Breath of Life,* and in it he claimed that the main difference between the whites—who lived in big cities, in crowded, overheated apartments—and Indians who lived outdoors in the fresh air was that from an early age the native people slept with their mouths closed and breathed through their noses. "There is no animal in nature excepting man, that sleeps with the mouth open; and with mankind, I believe the habit, which is not natural, is generally confined to civilized communities, where he is nurtured and raised amidst enervating luxuries and unnatural warmth. . . . The Savage infant, like the offspring of the brute, breathing the natural and wholesome air, generally from instinct, closes its mouth during its sleep; and in all cases of exception the mother rigidly (and cruelly, if necessary) enforces Nature's Law by pressing his lips together as it falls asleep until the habit is fixed for life."

Catlin suggested that his readers observe their sleeping children and see the expression of suffering on their faces and their tense muscles as they slept with mouths agape, and contrast it with an infant sleeping with closed mouth, whose facial expression was serene and calm. The smile on the face of the sleeping babe whose mouth is closed was overwhelming evidence that it was enjoying its sleep. Breathing through the mouth while asleep, Catlin claimed, caused snoring, a feeling of tiredness in the morning, headaches upon waking, and a strong desire to carry on sleeping. Moreover, he was convinced that breathing through the mouth while asleep caused increased susceptibility to illness, and even death. He concluded his book by suggesting that the sides of babies' cribs and cradles be inscribed with the three words "Shut Your Mouth," and it is hardly surprising that some years later he changed the book's title to "Shut Your Mouth and Save Your Life." His warnings preceded by at least a hundred years the modern descriptions of snoring as one of the clear signs of sleep disordered breathing.

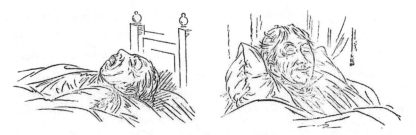

Sleeping with mouth open and mouth closed, from George Catlin's book
The Breath of Life, published in 1861

Catlin returned from his expeditions to the West with more than
five hundred paintings, items of Indian clothing, ritual artifacts, and
weapons, calling his collection Catlin's North American Portfolio and
preparing it for public exhibition. Although the first showings in New
York and Washington drew large and curious audiences, he did not succeed in persuading Congress to purchase the exhibition for the National
Museum. His preaching in support of Indian rights and against the plun-
der of their lands did not exactly heighten his popularity among the
members of Congress. Saddened by his failure, Catlin took his exhibition to Europe, where it was shown in England and France. Some years
later he lost most of his money, and the exhibition passed into the hands
of a wealthy American who stored it in his cellar. Disillusioned and desperate, Catlin continued his wanderings and spent a number of years in
the forests of South America, where he prospected for gold and painted
the native peoples. He died in 1872, seven years before Congress finally
purchased his Native American portfolio for the Smithsonian Institution, where it is housed to this day.

Although it should not be assumed that Catlin had met the ear,
nose, and throat specialist W. D. Wells, some years after the publication
of Catlin's book Wells described the cases of eighteen patients who had
difficulties breathing through the nose, and of these eight complained of
excessive daytime sleepiness. Surgery to improve their nasal breathing
also helped increase these patients' daytime wakefulness. In concluding
his article, Wells remarked that in many cases the patients were unaware
of the connection between difficulty in breathing through the nose and

daytime sleepiness. He suggested that physicians investigate their patients' sleeping habits, and added, "Though authors have failed to mark
this as a symptom of nasal stenosis, it is in fact an invariable one, if the
patient is not a mouth breather."

More than a century later, sleep laboratory examinations confirmed the assertions of Catlin and Wells by showing that people with
nose blockages indeed suffer from sleep disorders.

Doubts and Erroneous Diagnosis

The beginning of the twentieth century brought a dramatic change in attitudes toward sleep breathing disorders, which until then had been conspicuous in their absence from medical literature. Although here and
there one might come across a scientific article discussing Cheyne-
Stokes breathing in heart patients, the phenomenon of sleep disordered
breathing accompanied by loud snoring and followed by daytime sleepiness did not merit mention until the 1950s. Why sleep breathing disorders were ignored for so long was a result of the scientific approaches
and theories of the time regarding the nature of sleep in general, and also
the medical approach to the symptom of daytime sleepiness, which is
one of the most prominent signs of sleep disordered breathing.

Until the middle of the twentieth century, the scientific viewpoint
on sleep did not differ greatly from that of the two-thousand-year-old
school of thought introduced by Galen. Sleep was perceived as a passive state created by the disconnection of the brain from the rest of the
body parts and the external environment, or because of a slowing down
and inhibition of its activity—an approach to sleep that had existed since
the dawn of history. Alcmaeon, who lived in the sixth century B.C.E.,
claimed that sleep was brought on by the receding of the blood from the
vessels in the skin to the interior parts of the body, which caused immo-
bility and an absence of sensation. Some saw sleep as a result of changes
in the blood's characteristics, not its volume, or its distribution throughout the body. Cooling of the blood was the reason for sleep; a rise in its
temperature caused wakefulness. Aristotle explained sleep as a cooling

of the heart; Plato supplanted this idea with one suggesting cooling of the brain.

All these concepts survived for more than fifteen hundred years. The changes introduced by physicians and philosophers in the Middle Ages, the Renaissance, and even later were minimal. These experts' interest lay in the causes of the brain's isolation from the rest of the body, and there were those who explained this as variations in the brain's blood flow, the swelling of the lymph glands in the neck, and even as a physical disconnection between the nerve endings. Such an approach encouraged a view of sleep as essentially a physical state in which nothing happens, and consequently very few people took the trouble to engage in either sleep research or the study of sleep disorders.

The second reason for the sluggishness of research until the 1950s is linked to medical attitudes about excessive sleepiness. Physicians did not ascribe much importance to excessive daytime sleepiness unless it was related to a specific illness or damage to the central nervous system. It is therefore not surprising that at the beginning of the twentieth century daytime sleepiness was not even mentioned in the medical encyclopedias or reviews of sleep disorders. Even those articles dedicated to the subject were written in a slightly apologetic style. J. R. Gasquet, for example, in the introduction to his 1877 article, "On the Causes and Treatment of Drowsiness," first apologized to his readers for choosing to deal with "a subject of no great importance." Because daytime sleepiness characterized three different illnesses—narcolepsy, African sleeping sickness, and encephalitis lethargica—there was a prevalent belief that sleepiness was always linked to an organic illness, and these three illnesses are all involved with damage to the central nervous system. The discovery of narcolepsy had a particularly important bearing on medical attitudes toward excessive sleepiness.

Narcolepsy, first described by the French physician Jean-Baptiste-Edouard Gelineau in 1880, is characterized by frequent attacks of sleep during the day, accompanied by great muscular weakness. The impact of Gelineau's description of the illness was so great that, for many years after, the term "narcolepsy" was synonymous with a sleepy person, and almost every patient who complained of daytime sleepiness was diag-

nosed as "narcoleptic." Even Richard Caton titled his article describing
a patient with sleep disordered breathing "A Case of Narcolepsy." He
was not the only one to make the same mistake.

As its name suggests, African sleeping sickness is also connected
with severe disorders in the level of wakefulness. This illness was almost certainly known centuries before it was discovered by the Western
world. The first description of it appeared in *A History of the Berbers,* a
fourteenth-century book by 'Abd al-Rahman Ibn Khaldun. In it he wrote
of the sultan of what is today Mali, who suffered from "sleeping sickness" which in the end caused his death, and from the description and
symptoms of the illness we may assume it was African sleeping sickness.
Sleeping sickness, which is prevalent in Western and Central Africa, is
caused by the sting of the tsetse fly that carries the *Trypanosoma* parasite. After penetrating into the body, the parasite reproduces rapidly in
the blood and the lymph glands, crosses the blood-brain barrier, and in-
filtrates the brain tissue, where it causes serious neurological disorders.
Sleep disorders, in the form of excessive daytime sleepiness, and insomnia are the trademarks of the illness.

Even today, forty thousand to fifty thousand new cases of African
sleeping sickness are being discovered every year, and recently the situation has deteriorated even further as a result of the incessant armed con-
flicts in Africa. Electrophysiological recordings in African sleeping sickness patients show that in the first stage of the illness there is total
disorganization of the sleep-wakefulness rhythms, which indicates damage to the biological clock that oversees states of wakefulness. The more
advanced stages of the illness are marked by slow brain waves, which indicate sleep and sleepiness during the awake state.

The third disease characterized by excessive sleepiness, encephalitis lethargica, is also linked to brain damage. To this day we do not know
with any certainty the reasons for the outbreak of encephalitis that took
a toll of approximately 5 million victims throughout the world between
1916 and 1930. The mysterious illness appeared out of nowhere in the
winter of 1916, and those who contracted it usually experienced high
fever, hallucinations, impaired vision, and severe sleep disorders. As a
result of the extraordinary combination of symptoms, the patients were

initially diagnosed with a variety of illnesses, from schizophrenia through Parkinson's disease. Constantin von Economo, a Romanian-born Austrian psychiatrist, was the first to pinpoint the factor common to all the cases. In May 1916 he published an article on the newly discovered disease, which he called encephalitis lethargica or sleeping sickness. In the article he wrote that the thread connecting all the cases of encephalitis was the serious sleep disorders, which manifested themselves in the form of excessive sleepiness that lasted for weeks and months, or a total lack of sleep that ended in death.

The disease's effect on sleep was dramatic: approximately one-third of the patients fell asleep for extended periods, and it was impossible to wake them. The majority died while still asleep. Some suffered from the opposite symptom—a total inability to fall asleep even with the help of drugs. A small number of patients sank into a sleep something like Rip van Winkle's, from which they awoke forty or fifty years later. In the 1950s, Oliver Sacks, the London-born American neurologist, found some of these patients in a New York institution for the chronically sick and treated them with L-dopa (levodopa), which awakened them from their endless sleep. Unfortunately, the end of the story was a sad one: Sacks was forced to stop the wonder drug treatment because of the serious side effects it produced. Robin Williams and Robert De Niro commemorated Sacks and one of his patients in the movie *Awakenings*.

Not only did von Economo discover the common denominator of all the cases, but he also found the reasons for sleep disorders. When he examined the brains of patients who had died from the disease, in all of them he found signs of brain damage caused by the inflammation. When the disease was characterized by serious sleep disorders, the damage was always located in the same area of the brain, very close to the hypothalamus, which controls activities like eating, drinking, sex, and the function of the autonomic nervous system, among other things. When the clinical symptoms included excessive sleepiness, the damage was located in the posterior part of the hypothalamus, and when lack of sleep was one of the symptoms, the damage was in the anterior area. Based on his observations, von Economo concluded that the area adjacent to the hypothalamus was linked to the control of sleep and, for reasons that were unclear, that the disease affected this particular area, which led to the serious sleep disorders. Strangely, however, at the end of the 1920s, encephalitis lethargica vanished as suddenly and mysteriously as it had appeared.

From the history of these three diseases, it is easy to understand why severe excessive daytime sleepiness became a hallmark of encephalitis or other organic illness. Hundreds of scientific articles published at the beginning of the twentieth century on African sleeping sickness, narcolepsy, and encephalitis lethargica left no doubt regarding the organic source of excessive daytime sleepiness. The widely held view was that people did not just fall asleep during the day for no particular reason, or against their will, even if they had serious disorders in their nighttime sleep. Rather, it had to be because they suffered from a disease that damaged the brain.

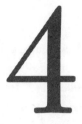

Rediscovery of the Pickwickian Patient

The only exceptions to the theory holding that sleepiness is always a symptom of central nervous system damage, or disease, were the obese sleepyheads. As in the nineteenth century, the combination of obesity and sleepiness, often in the most embarrassing circumstances, captured the attention of twentieth-century physicians who were lovers of Dickens and who occasionally "rediscovered" the Pickwickian syndrome.

To this day the most oft-quoted article on the subject is one written by Sidney Burwell and his colleagues in 1956. The article, titled "Extreme Obesity Associated with Alveolar Hypoventilation—A Pickwickian Syndrome," describes the case of a sleepy, obese patient as follows.

> He was a fifty-one year old business executive who entered the hospital because of obesity, fatigue and somnolence. This patient reported that he had been overweight all his remembered life and for many years had weighed approximately 100 kg. When this weight was maintained, he was alert, vigorous and able to work long hours. . . . As the patient gained weight his symptoms appeared and became worse. . . . He had often fallen asleep while carrying on his daily routine. . . . Finally an experience which indicated the severity of his disability led him to seek hospital care. The patient was

37

accustomed to playing poker once a week and on this crucial
occasion he was dealt a hand of three aces and two kings.
This hand is called a "full house." *Because he had dropped off
to sleep he failed to take advantage of this opportunity.* A few
days later he entered the Peter Bent Brigham Hospital. [Em-
phasis in the original]

Although this article is frequently cited as the first medical description of sleep apnea syndrome, it is not so. The case description
makes it almost certain that the card player suffered from sleep disordered breathing, but Burwell and his colleagues do not discuss the patient's sleep and do not ascribe his drowsiness to a sleep disorder.
Rather, they explain that the patient's excess weight made his breathing
inefficient, which caused a rise in the carbon dioxide level in his blood,
resulting in drowsiness. (For a number of years following the article's appearance the sleepiness experienced by such patients was ascribed to
"carbon dioxide poisoning.") Furthermore, as we have seen, Caton,
Morrison, and others had described similar cases earlier. It is difficult to
say why Burwell's article became so popular, but it may have something
to do with the title, which crowned the syndrome "Pickwickian" (although the paper contained no mention of all those who had used the
same coinage for the combination of obesity and drowsiness many years
earlier). There is also the memorable story of the card player falling
asleep in the middle of a game while holding an almost unbeatable hand,
which provides a piquant and distinctive medical anecdote, although in
this too Burwell was preceded by Morrison. Whatever the reason, the article's effect was enormous. The term "Pickwickian syndrome" was enthusiastically adopted by the medical community, and dozens of similar
cases of Pickwickian patients were reported in the 1960s and '70s.

The first sleep researchers, who began their work in the sixties in
the wake of articles on dream sleep by Nathaniel Kleitman and Eugene
Aserinsky in 1953 and embarked on the study of sleep with the help of
electrophysiological measuring instruments, totally ignored the existence of obese and drowsy patients. The first years of modern sleep research were characterized by normative research that studied the sleep

of people of various ages or of those with a variety of illnesses. Researchers at the time focused on narcoleptics, insomniacs, and the sleep of mentally ill patients with depression and schizophrenia. Drowsy patients were of no interest, and so the Pickwickians became solely the province of internists and pulmonary specialists, who attributed the patients' drowsiness to their blood gas levels, a subject with which the sleep researchers were unfamiliar and in which they probably had no interest. Even when the first descriptions of sleep disordered breathing in Pickwickian patients appeared, they initially left no impression on the sleep research community and for many years lay unnoticed between the pages of medical journals.

An Internist with an Interest in Brain Waves

The first physiological recordings in sleeping Pickwickian patients were conducted in 1960 at the Ludolf Krehl Clinic of the Heidelberg University Hospital, and a year later at the National Institutes of Health in Bethesda, Maryland. The significance of these observations remained unnoticed by almost all who came later, and their primary importance has so far failed to gain the recognition they deserve.

Werner Gerardy completed his medical studies at the University of Mainz, Germany, in 1951. Two years later he received an appointment to the internal medicine department at the Heidelberg University Hospital, where he began his research. His subject was quite out of the ordinary among internists: how internal diseases affect the brain's electrical activity. Measurement of the brain's electrical activity, recorded in the form of electroencephalograms (EEG), was a subject usually found in the professional territory of neurologists. As some of the diseases in which Gerardy was interested were also characterized by autonomic nervous system activity, the hospital technicians made a number of adjustments to the electroencephalograph machine so that it would be able to record breathing and pulse rates at the same time as brain waves. Gerardy had no special interest in Pickwickian patients: he was studying people with diseases of the liver and blood vessels, in whom he looked for symptoms of disorders in the electrical function of the brain. It was pure chance that led him to conduct a sleep recording, the first in medical history, on a Pickwickian patient.

Professor Dieter Herberg, head of the internal medicine department in which Gerardy worked, conducted morning rounds in his department every day and his progress was marked by a long train of young doctors who followed in his wake, hanging on to his every word—a familiar sight on hospital rounds. On one of the professor's rounds, attended by Gerardy, they came across a patient lying in bed, not breathing and completely "blue" from lack of oxygen. The entire group rushed to his bedside, convinced that he had died, only to see—to their great astonishment—that he suddenly renewed his breathing very loudly, and the signs of cyanosis vanished as if they had never existed. A check of the patient's records revealed that he had been hospitalized because of reduced work capacity and, apart from frequent headaches upon waking, there was no apparent reason for his fainting attacks. To investigate the cause of the headaches, Gerardy was instructed to conduct an electroencephalogram examination, as usual in such cases. Happily, he did the recordings on the electroencephalograph that had been adapted for his research by the addition of channels to measure breathing and pulse rates.

According to usual practice, the brain wave examination was conducted during the day and lasted for about an hour. The results, as Gerardy described later with great exactitude, were surprising: "Approximately ten minutes after the commencement of recording, the patient was sleeping deeply. Here, periodic breathing was observed with short suspensions with the tongue sometimes falling back at the onset of each suspension so that there was no airflow, despite the increased movements of the thorax. Then the patient woke up suddenly, the tongue moved forward and a second, or a second and a half later, the first breath appeared. The heart rate during the suspension of breathing became slower and slower, but was greatly accelerated with renewal of breathing." Gerardy and his colleagues then examined another Pickwickian patient, and with him, too, they observed the same phenomenon. Both patients, who were employed as clerks by the postal authority, were afflicted with excessive obesity and a tendency to fall asleep "under any conditions and at any time." Both showed a great improvement in their sleep and level of wakefulness after losing weight.

Gerardy, Herberg, and another researcher named Hans Manfred Kuhn described their findings in the first report on a sleep recording in Pickwickian patients, published in Germany in 1960. Their explanation for the suspension of breathing during sleep was no different from the views then prevailing regarding the causes of breathing disorders and drowsiness in Pickwickian patients: because the patients' breathing was shallow and inefficient, their blood held a high concentration of carbon dioxide, and as a result the sensitivity of the breathing center in the brain stem to changes in blood gas levels was reduced. This in turn caused the control of breathing in obese patients to shift to the carotid bodies, which act to vary breathing in accordance with the blood oxygen level, not that of carbon dioxide. As the control mechanism of the carotid bodies is less refined, any reduction in the blood oxygen saturation level also caused the activation of the arousal mechanism in the brain stem, and consequently an awakening from sleep. This, the authors claimed, was also the reason for the complaints of some Pickwickian patients that they frequently awoke from their sleep, although the researchers did not make the connection between the patients' daytime drowsiness and the frequent disruptions of their sleep. Like others, they assumed that the source of daytime sleepiness was in "carbon dioxide poisoning."

Moreover, Gerardy and his colleagues did not ascribe importance to the fact that at the onset of an apnea, the Pickwickian patient's tongue fell backward, blocking the pharynx, and that the renewal of breathing was accompanied by a forward movement of the tongue. They viewed this purely as a sign of deepening sleep. Only later did it become clear that this blockage of the pharynx plays a central role in sleep apnea syndrome.

Gerardy's brief research career ended in 1962, when he left Heidelberg for an appointment as head of the internal medicine department at another hospital. The burden of his clinical duties as a department head left him insufficient time to continue with active medical research. Now in his eighties, Gerardy still practices medicine at a rehabilitation facility where he works mainly with cardiac patients.

Awakenings or Falling Asleep?

Two years after Gerardy's article was published in Germany, Daniel Drachman and Robert Gumnit of the United States National Institutes of Health published an article in the journal of the American Neurological Society titled "Periodic Alteration of Consciousness in the Pickwickian Syndrome." Gumnit, a researcher in the neurophysiology and electroencephalography laboratories at the National Institutes of Health, had a great interest in the brain waves of epileptic patients and patients who had lost consciousness as a result of a blow to the head. But he was also curious about the tendency of Pickwickian patients to frequently fall asleep and awaken during the day. To study this phenomenon, he and Drachman conducted recordings of brain waves, breathing movements, the saturation levels of oxygen and the concentration of carbon dioxide in the blood of a drowsy female Pickwickian patient. The patient was fifty-seven and had been hospitalized because of an uncontrollable tendency to fall asleep during the day that had gone on for several years. She was an ice cream vendor whose enthusiasm for sampling her wares had led to a weight increase of twenty kilograms in the space of three months, and she tipped the scales at some one hundred kilos. Drachman and Gumnit noted that, despite her falling asleep numerous times during the day and immediately at night, her sleep was restless. Moreover, people who had observed her testified that she tended to choke and suffocate as she slept.

Like Gerardy and his colleagues, Drachman and Gumnit tested the patient's daytime sleep. So long as her brain waves showed that she was awake, her breathing functions and blood gas levels were normal, but the moment her brain waves showed that she had fallen asleep, her breathing ceased and the oxygen saturation level in her blood dropped to a minimum of almost 50 percent. And then, about half a minute later, the patient awakened again and started breathing, and the oxygen saturation level in her blood rose, only for her to stop breathing again after a few seconds, and so on. As in Gerardy's patients, her pulse rate also varied—from 50 beats per minute during the apneas to 140 when she awoke. The patient's main complaint was that she fell asleep numerous times during the day, and during the examination Drachman and Gumnit found that she fell asleep, for short periods of about half a minute each, approximately two hundred times a day. We know today that the patient's true condition was exactly the opposite: she did not, in fact, fall asleep two hundred times but *awakened* from sleep two hundred times. Drachman and Gumnit knew of Gerardy's article, and like them they explained the Pickwickian patients' excessive sleepiness as carbon dioxide "poisoning."

As for the ice-cream-loving patient, a strict diet of six hundred calories per day for six days helped her shed twenty kilograms and brought about the almost complete disappearance of her daytime sleepiness.

In being the first to conduct recordings of brain waves, pulse rate, and breathing functions in sleeping Pickwickian patients, Gerardy and colleagues and Drachman and Gumnit broke new ground in sleep research. Additionally, they identified the suspensions of breathing during sleep, noted the tongue falling backward during apneas, and even documented the effect of apneas on the saturation level of oxygen in the blood and the pulse rate. Furthermore, both groups of researchers found clear evidence that the patients slept restlessly at night and awakened frequently. Researchers who came after them remained largely unaware of the importance of both these articles, possibly because both studies were conducted during the daytime and not at night, or because the articles' titles did not accurately reflect their content, or because in both cases the examining physicians were not part of the sleep research community. Whatever the reason, both reports were milestones in the modern history of sleep apnea syndrome. And four years later, sleep researchers did learn about the crazy sleep of Pickwickian patients. The man responsible for this was a German neurologist who showed a great interest in the physiological changes that accompanied the process of falling asleep.

The Ski Resort Symposium

Wolfgang Kuhl, who had studied medicine in Freiburg and specialized in neurology, was interested in the relationship between the electrical activity of the brain and states of consciousness. In his early studies, which he conducted in conjunction with geneticists, he investigated the possibility that human brain wave patterns are hereditary. He later turned his attention to the characteristics of the brain's electrical activity during the transition from wakefulness to sleep, and how these changes are reflected in the subjective experiences of human beings. All this prepared him well for the study of Pickwickian patients' sleep.

In 1960, Kuhl was appointed director of a laboratory for the study of brain waves at Freiburg University's department of neurophysiology. The department was headed by Richard Jung, one of the pioneers of neurophysiology in Germany, who was extremely interested in the Pickwickian syndrome. Jung had been impressed by the work of Bulow and Ingvar on breathing instability during the falling-asleep process, and he suggested that Kuhl conduct nighttime sleep recordings on Pickwickian patients. He assumed that in these patients the breathing instability would continue through the night, and Kuhl's recordings indeed showed that the moment Pickwickian patients fell asleep they stopped breathing and immediately awakened and renewed their breathing, only to fall asleep again and stop breathing. But in contrast to their predecessors, who did not connect the sleep disorder with daytime sleepiness, Kuhl and Jung correctly concluded that the disorder in the Pickwickian patients' daytime level of wakefulness lay in the recurring interruption in the course of their sleep, and was not because of carbon dioxide poisoning. Another difference was the stage on which Kuhl and Jung's findings were presented, which turned their work into a noteworthy achievement in the history of sleep research. Kuhl presented his paper at one of the European Neurological Society's annual conferences, which are known as the "skiing conferences."

The European Neurological Society has a long-standing tradition of holding scientific conferences on the study of brain waves at famous ski resorts, where the participants combine scientific lectures with speeding down the piste. The first conference was held in 1959 at Saint Moritz, one of Switzerland's more glittering resorts, and since then the participants have gathered at a different European ski resort each year. The day usually begins at eight-thirty, when the participants head off to enjoy the ski slopes until late afternoon, and at about four o'clock the scientific part of the conference gets under way and lasts until the evening. Unlike most scientific conferences in recent years at which the proceedings and lectures are given in English, which has become the lingua franca of science, at the first skiing conferences the neurologists presented their studies in their native tongues. The younger members, who were fluent in several languages, translated the proceedings into English when necessary. Roger Broughton of Ottawa, who today is one of the world's leading sleep researchers, told me that the lectures in English translation were often immeasurably better than in their source language.

Kuhl presented the findings of his recordings of the nighttime sleep of a Pickwickian patient at the skiing conference held at Oberstdorf in the German Alps in 1964. Although Drachman and Gumnit's article had been published in a respected neurology journal two years earlier, it had not gained much attention, so this was actually the first time that neurologists with a specific interest in sleep were exposed to the subject of sleep disordered breathing in Pickwickian syndrome patients.

It is not difficult to understand the great interest aroused by the case in question. Pickwickian syndrome, which had been the exclusive property of pulmonary specialists and internists, was presented by Kuhl in a totally different light. His recordings clearly showed that the syndrome originated not in shallow and inefficient breathing or heart disease, but in a disorder in the normal course of sleep—a subject that was in the field of research interest of some of those present at the lecture. And indeed, in Kuhl's audience at Oberstdorf were two people who immediately grasped the great importance and clinical significance of his findings: Henri Gastaut, head of the Neurobiological Research Unit in Marseilles, and his former student, Elio Lugaresi from Bologna. Many years after the conference, Kuhl recalled that immediately after his lecture Gastaut and Lugaresi had a heated and protracted discussion in French—apparently on his findings—of which Kuhl did not understand a single word.

Gastaut, whose research on the electrical activity of the brain in epileptics had made him a world-renowned neurologist, ordered sleep recordings on Pickwickian patients as soon as he returned to Marseilles. The task was given to Bernard Duron, a young researcher well-versed in respiratory function and neurophysiology, who immediately went to work. The first Pickwickian patient to spend a night attached to the recording instruments in the Marseilles sleep laboratory stopped breathing in his sleep, just as Kuhl had reported at the skiing conference. But in contrast to Kuhl and Jung's findings that the source of the disorder was in a dysfunction of the brain's respiratory center, the Marseilles group's conclusion was completely different. According to Duron's sleep recordings, the cause of the apneas was in the blockage of the upper airways during sleep. In other words, the respiratory center continued working but the patient did not manage to breathe because his airways were blocked. How did they reach this conclusion? In contrast to Kuhl and Jung, who attached sensors for measuring thorax contractions to their Pickwickian patient and tested the concentration of carbon dioxide in the exhaled air, Duron tested the airflow in the nostrils and mouth and also the movements of the thorax. In this way he was able to determine that, despite the airflow having ceased, there was no complete suspension of respiratory muscle activity and thorax movement, both of which continued working with even greater intensity to unblock the upper airways. Therefore, where Kuhl and Jung ascribed the disorder to a disruption of respiratory center activity during sleep, Gastaut and his colleagues attributed it to a blockage of the airways. It is no wonder that Duron later became a professor of pulmonary medicine.

Sleep recording in several more patients led the Marseilles group to distinguish between three types of apneas, or suspensions of breathing, during sleep: an obstructive apnea in which there is a suspension of airflow in the nose and mouth, despite continued energetic activity of the respiratory muscles; an apnea with a central origin, in which there is a suspension of respiratory muscle activity together with a suspension of airflow; and a mixed apnea, which starts as a central apnea and ends as an obstructive apnea. It later became clear that in the majority of patients, the apneas were of the obstructive or the mixed type, while central apneas mainly characterize patients with diseases of the central nervous system. Carlo A. Tassinari, a young neurologist from Bologna who was also in frequent contact with Lugaresi and his group, participated in these pioneering sleep studies of Pickwickian patients.

Jung and Kuhl published their first article on breathing disorders in the sleep of Pickwickian patients in a collection of articles presented at an international symposium on sleep mechanisms held at the University of Zurich in September 1964. In it they described three cases in which, during the night, they recorded brain waves, thorax movements, and carbon dioxide levels in the exhaled air. The recordings showed apneas lasting for twenty to forty seconds and appearing cyclically. Each apnea ended in an awakening, which was evidenced by the brain wave recording. In each of the three patients a weight reduction of ten to twenty kilograms brought about a significant improvement in sleep breathing functions and daytime sleepiness, even though the apneas did not disappear completely. Interestingly, Kuhl and Jung cited the articles by Gerardy and colleagues and Drachman and Gumnit, but did not discuss their findings at all. They apparently did not ascribe any particular importance to these articles and did not study them in depth.

It is hard to say whether Kuhl and Jung's paper left a great impression on the participants in the Zurich symposium. The physician who summed up the symposium from the internist's point of view did not even mention their findings, and neither did Giuseppe Moruzzi, one of the greatest neurophysiologists of the time, who summarized the symposium from the neurophysiology standpoint.

The Sleep Laboratory in the Bathroom

The third aspect of the modern story of sleep apnea syndrome is deeply rooted in the neurology clinic at the University of Bologna, which proudly bears the name "Europe's first university." Elio Lugaresi and Giorgio Coccagna, two young neurologists from Bologna, also took part in the 1964 skiing conference at Oberstdorf, where they listened attentively to Kuhl's lecture. They, too, were not newcomers to the field of sleep research and as soon as they heard Kuhl's observations they eagerly returned to the laboratory to examine the phenomenon for themselves.

Influenced by the discovery of rapid eye movement (REM) sleep by Aserinsky and Kleitman in 1953, Lugaresi had set up a sleep research laboratory in Bologna for neurological patients. Every night, a large bathroom that did daytime duty serving the hospital doctors was turned into a sophisticated sleep laboratory. Every evening, Lugaresi and his colleagues dragged the bed and recording instruments into the bathroom and then led the patient inside for his or her night's sleep. The "bathroom" recordings certainly provided some exciting results.

In their first study Lugaresi and his colleagues conducted sleep recordings on patients with "restless legs syndrome" during sleep. They showed that these patients display periodic involuntary leg movements while asleep, with the number of movements running as high as several hundred a night, a condition they termed "nocturnal myoclonus." Their unique contribution to nocturnal myoclonus was to demonstrate that it was not an epileptic disorder, as suggested by the English neurologist Sir Charles Symmonds, but a sleep-related disorder. Later it was shown that this frequent "kicking" during sleep caused sleep interruptions, so that the patients complained of insomnia or lack of sleep.

These experiments set the stage in Bologna for sleep recordings of Pickwickian patients, which quickly verified the Freiburg and Marseilles findings. Moreover, the Bologna group's findings even supported those of the Marseilles researchers that the source of the sleep disorder in Pickwickian patients was a blockage of the airways, and not a dysfunction in the activity of the brain's respiratory center. Like the Marseilles group, Lugaresi and his colleagues also distinguished between obstructive, central, and mixed apneas. Later, Daniel Kurtz and Jean Krieger of Strasbourg added a further type of sleep disordered breathing, hypopnea, or a partial suspension of breathing. These cases show a reduction in the airflow through the nose or mouth of as much as two-thirds of the normal level, but without a total suspension. Like a full apnea, hypopnea ends with a brief awakening reaction and a slight drop in the oxygen saturation level. Today there is no differentiation between full and partial suspensions of breathing, and both are defined as sleep disordered breathing.

Lugaresi and his colleagues took a further step in the investigation of sleep breathing disorders in Pickwickian patients, and they did so with the assistance of the wife of Coccagna, Lugaresi's research collaborator. Paola Verucci Coccagna was an anesthetist with wide experience in monitoring the vital signs of anesthetized patients. With her husband's encouragement she joined the group in order to test, for the first time, how sleep apneas affect patients' systemic and pulmonary blood pressure.

Monitoring the blood pressure of sleeping Pickwickian patients revealed some dramatic findings: the apneas and the renewal of breathing caused extreme variations in both systemic and pulmonary blood pressure. Blood pressure dropped at the onset of the apnea and rose dramatically when breathing was resumed, together with a brief awakening from sleep. With the apneas occurring throughout the course of sleep and variations in blood pressure accompanying each of them, Pickwickian patients showed extreme rises and falls in blood pressure every minute during their sleep. Immediately after discovering that sleep apneas cause such wide variations in blood pressure, Lugaresi decided that the time was ripe for his cardiologist and pulmonary specialist colleagues to participate in researching the syndrome. His invitation to observe the sleep of Pickwickian patients was accepted, and while his new colleagues were deeply impressed by the nocturnal spectacle of seeing a patient suffocate in his sleep hundreds of times a night, they did not view it as a subject suitable for research.

Many years later, when the medical community had become aware of the challenge of apnea during sleep, I asked Lugaresi how he explained the indifference his colleagues displayed toward the syndrome in the 1960s and '70s. He attributed it to the fact that at the time, only observations published in "the medical holy writ," such as the *New England Journal of Medicine, The Lancet,* and the *British Medical Journal* were legitimate subjects for research. Observations that did not merit publication in the leading medical journals gained no attention whatsoever. Even actually seeing the phenomenon did not convince Lugaresi's colleagues of the syndrome's importance—and they were not the only ones.

The Tracheostomy Dilemma

Lugaresi's observations on the dramatic rise in blood pressure during apneas in sleep mandated a different approach to the phenomenon. It was now clear that this was not simply a strange medical episode but a disorder that called for treatment, and even aggressive treatment. Until this time the only treatment for Pickwickian patients was a reduction in weight, but losing weight was no simple thing for such obese people. Even when it was clear that a significant loss of body weight considerably improved their sleep, only a few patients were capable of losing weight and persevering with a reducing diet for an extended period. Gastaut's and Lugaresi's observations on upper airway blockages in Pickwickian patients suggested an alternative treatment by means of bypassing the blockage. To bypass a pharyngeal blockage, an alternative opening had to be made in the trachea, using a procedure called tracheostomy. Patients could close the opening in their neck with a suitable stopper during the day, and at night they could remove it to enable normal breathing. Tracheostomy is no small thing, leaving the patient open to risk of infection and even possible damage to speech. It is hardly surprising that Lugaresi and his colleagues hesitated and deliberated long and hard about whether tracheostomy for the Pickwickian patients in their care was justified. Moreover, they were not entirely convinced that the procedure would improve the patients' condition. Their findings indicated that it was entirely possible that the upper airway blockage was also related to a certain laxity in the respiratory muscles' activity as a result of a disruption of the respiratory center.

But chance intervened, bringing with it a radical change in their position, and once again it was Kuhl who changed the course of things. One of his Pickwickian patients had sunk into a protracted coma as a result of what was diagnosed as severe carbon dioxide poisoning. To save him from this desperate situation, all that remained for the doctors to do was perform a tracheostomy. To their astonishment, the patient awakened from his coma immediately after the procedure and appeared to have made a complete recovery from not only his sleep disordered breathing but also his attacks of daytime sleepiness. This case convinced Kuhl that Gastaut and Lugaresi were right about the sleep breathing disorder in Pickwickian patients, and that the source of the disorder was blockage of the upper airways and not a disruption in the activity of the respiratory center. The tracheostomy seemed to have solved the problem completely. On hearing about Kuhl's case, Lugaresi and his colleagues managed to convince the staff of the Bologna surgical department to perform emergency tracheostomy procedures on the Pickwickian patients in their care. Within a short time six patients underwent the procedure, and on the first night after surgery all of them showed that the apneas had completely disappeared, together with the daytime sleepiness. Furthermore, post-treatment general and pulmonary blood pressure recordings showed a significant improvement, and pathological signs in two patients disappeared from their sleep electrocardiogram recordings.

Convinced of the importance of their new findings in Pickwickian patients, Lugaresi and Giorgio Coccagna decided to organize a scientific conference in Bologna dedicated to sleep disorders. The conference was held in 1967 and became the first of a series on the subject, and it drew sleep researchers from all over the world, including William Dement and Allan Rechtschaffen, the pioneers of modern sleep research in the United States, Gastaut and Pierre Passouant from France, Ian Oswald from Scotland, Bedrich Roth from Prague, and Yasuo Hishikawa from Japan—who crossed Asia by rail on the Trans-Siberian Express to save the price of an air ticket from Japan to Italy, and after the conference did advanced studies at Kuhl's laboratory in Freiburg and then became Japan's first researcher in the field of sleep disorders. Today it is clear that the Bologna conference laid the cornerstone of the field of sleep medicine, and all its participants became key figures in the study of sleep and its disorders. Only few of those who attended, however, rushed back to their laboratories to study sleep disordered breathing.

William Dement from Stanford, who established the first clinic in the United States for diagnosis of sleep disorders, admitted that he completely missed the importance of the test findings in the sleep of Pickwickian patients reported in Bologna. The main thrust of his work at the time was directed toward narcolepsy, and he was not the only one to remain indifferent to the sleep of Pickwickians. A study of the programs of the first scientific conferences of the European Sleep Research Society, which was founded in 1965, does not reveal any articles on the Pickwickian syndrome except for two further case descriptions. Brief reports on sleep recordings conducted on the odd Pickwickian patient appeared here and there in the medical literature, but they contained no innovations. In Prague, for example, sleep recordings were conducted on a small number of Pickwickian patients who were referred for testing by an obesity clinic. Dr. Sona Nevsimalova, who today is the head of Charles

University's department of neurology in Prague, participated in the first
sleep recordings of Pickwickian patients, and explained the lack of interest in their sleep as a result of most everyone being deeply immersed
in study of the narcolepsy syndrome. Even Kuhl did not continue his
study of sleep in Pickwickian patients beyond his groundbreaking sleep
recordings. Interest in the subject amounted to sporadic sleep studies of
Pickwickian patients in France, Switzerland, Germany, and Italy. Lugaresi and his colleagues, and Duron and Tassinari in Marseilles, were
the only ones who continued the methodical study of the sleep of patients who stopped breathing while asleep. Gastaut was not interested
anymore because apneas during sleep had been shown to have no relation to epilepsy, which was his particular field of interest.

Five years later, in 1972, the Bologna group organized another scientific conference devoted to the subject of the Pickwickian syndrome,
this one titled Hypersomnia and Periodic Breathing. This conference
was held at the Italian resort of Rimini, and papers were presented on
sleep disordered breathing, sleep recordings of patients, and treatment
using tracheostomy. This was the first time an attempt was made to distinguish between the different types of Pickwickian patients. Douglas
Carroll from Baltimore specified no fewer than ten different types of
Pickwickian syndromes. One of them, which he termed the Gastaut's
type, was characterized by "obesity with hypersomnia (which is excessive sleepiness) secondary to sleep loss, secondary to nocturnal upper
airway obstruction." Later Carroll reduced the number of Pickwickian
subtypes to two—with and without hypersomnia. In 1973, Dement and
Christian Guilleminault, working at Stanford University, showed that
hypersomnia associated nocturnal upper airway obstruction occurred
also in people with normal weight.

The papers from the Rimini conference were published in a special edition of *Bulletin de Physiopathologie Respiratoire,* a little-known
journal that a few years later ceased to exist, but in the meantime had a
decisive effect on the professional path taken by at least two of the eminent researchers of sleep apnea syndrome.

5

Western Innovations

Sleep research is one of the few scientific fields that can be traced with great accuracy to a particular starting point, after which things were totally different. Scientific sleep research began in 1953, when Nathaniel Kleitman and his student Eugene Aserinsky first described dream sleep, or rapid eye movement sleep, in a now-classic article published in *Science*.

During the 1960s, the few researchers engaged in studying the sleep of people suffering from sleep disorders focused on narcolepsy. In 1967, three independent groups from three continents—Rechtschaffen and Dement in the United States, Passouant and his colleagues in France, and Hishikawa and his colleagues in Japan—reported a surprising discovery concerning narcolepsy and REM sleep. In persons with normal sleep, REM sleep first appears about ninety minutes after they fall asleep. In narcoleptic patients, by contrast, REM sleep begins immediately after falling asleep. This discovery fired the imaginations of numerous sleep researchers, who hoped that they would be able to diagnose many more illnesses, such as schizophrenia and depression, according to sleep patterns. Except for the lone article published by Gumnit and Drachman describing the daytime sleep findings in the ice-cream-loving Pickwickian patient, almost nothing was done in the United States on the subject of sleep disordered breathing until the mid-1970s.

I completed my Ph.D. in psychology in 1973 at the University of

Florida sleep laboratory in Gainesville, under the tutelage of Bernie Webb, one of the founding fathers of modern sleep research in the United States. At the time there were only 150 to 200 people working on sleep research throughout the United States, and not one was engaged in the laboratory diagnosis of sleep disorders. The few sleep laboratories doing clinical examinations tested the effect of drugs on sleep patterns in normal humans, or in those with insomnia. It was, in fact, drug companies that first discovered the potential of laboratory sleep recordings, and they consequently invested vast sums in it. Instead of relying on patients' reports on the efficacy of a drug, they were able to receive a professional opinion written by sleep "experts" that was based on objective measurements. Of course, the actual sleep laboratory test of a specific drug later became a superb sales promotion tool.

On completion of my doctoral studies in Florida, I went to the University of California, San Diego, for post-doctorate studies in the department of psychiatry. The sleep laboratory was located in the hospital there, and in 1974 I came across many people suffering from insomnia or narcolepsy—as well as my first sleep apnea patient.

He was a very obese man who had been admitted due to complications resulting from hypertension. Oddly enough, his referral to the sleep laboratory was on the initiative of the nurses in the department where he was hospitalized, and there were two reasons for this. First, they reported that the patient was in a permanent state of sleep—while lying down, sitting, and even standing—and, second, his extremely loud snoring kept the rest of the patients awake and had forced the nurses to put him in a room by himself. We agreed enthusiastically to their request, because at the time we seized any opportunity to prove to the medical fraternity—which was totally indifferent to sleep research—that sleep recordings were of clinical importance. The majority of clinicians dismissed the possibility that there might be any significance in sleep recordings and viewed what went on in sleep laboratories as just another kind of research that was conducted, by its nature, at rather inconvenient hours. There had to be a very special reason for doctors to agree to spend their nights in a laboratory observing the brain waves of a sleeping person.

We were aware of the reports in the literature, especially those from Bologna and Marseilles, containing evidence that obese patients tended to experience respiratory disorders during sleep, so we decided to conduct some additional tests. Apart from the standard recordings of brain waves, muscle tonus, and eye movements, we tested the activity of the thoracic muscles and airflow in the nostrils. The results were amazing.

The moment the recording instruments showed that the patient had fallen asleep, he stopped breathing for a full fifty seconds. The correlation between falling asleep and cessation of breathing was remarkably accurate. The patient stopped breathing at the very moment that the alpha brain waves denoting wakefulness were replaced by the theta waves of sleep stage 1. Although it was clearly evident that he made a supreme effort to renew his breathing, something appeared to be stuck in his throat, blocking the flow of air. The patient was literally fighting for his life, lifting his whole body from the bed in an effort to renew the flow of air. Suddenly, the "blockage" was freed and he began to breathe again, at the same time emitting loud snores, but a few seconds later he stopped breathing again. The recording showed that he had begun to breathe only after the brain waves indicating wakefulness had appeared; at the very moment he had fallen asleep again, he had stopped breathing. This cycle of apneas, a brief awakening, renewal of breathing, then another apnea, recurred throughout the night. The patient suffered hundreds of apneas, each of which was terminated by a brief awakening and the emission of loud snores. In the morning we counted more than 450 suspensions of breathing, each one having lasted for thirty to fifty seconds.

Because the test results were so dramatic, we asked the patient to return to sleep in the laboratory during the day so that we could present this medical marvel to the hospital staff. When we repeated the test, the doctors huddled around the recording instruments were unable to conceal their amazement at the drama unfolding before them in the adjoining bedroom. Some even expressed fear that the patient might die in his sleep, as though they were witnessing an isolated and extraordinary example of sleep, and suggested that we awaken him. It was difficult to convince them that the patient had slept this way for many years.

I do not know what became of our patient. Although the case

caused great excitement and became a topic of conversation in the hospital's corridors and cafeteria for a few days, it did not greatly change the laboratory's work. We continued to test the effects of sleeping drugs and study biological rhythms. Until the end of 1974, when I returned to Israel, we saw no more patients with sleep apnea syndrome. Surprisingly, fifteen years later I was seeing three or four new apnea patients a week.

Other sleep researchers had similar experiences. Bill Orr went to the University of Oklahoma Medical School in 1973 after completing his doctoral studies in sleep research. He set up an improvised sleep laboratory in a small, crowded room allocated by the Oklahoma City Presbyterian Hospital. He borrowed surplus equipment from the hospital's various departments, and by chance the room serving as his sleep laboratory was located opposite the intensive care unit. One night he received a visit from Dr. N. K. Imes, head of the ICU, who popped in to find out more about the mysterious nocturnal goings-on next door. Orr, of course, was eager to tell Imes about what he was doing and about the wonders of sleep research. Imes told him about an odd phenomenon of patients from his unit who stopped breathing while asleep, adding that on that very night such a patient had been admitted. Orr enthusiastically took the opportunity to observe his first sleep apnea patient, and subsequently from 1973 to 1974 Orr and Imes examined numerous ICU patients who suffered from the same phenomenon. The relatively large number of patients with this condition led them to conclude that this was no rarity but rather a very common disorder—although their conclusion did not gain much support at the time.

Orr, Imes, and their colleagues in the ear, nose, and throat department of Oklahoma City Presbyterian Hospital were also among the first in North America to perform a tracheostomy on a sleep apnea syndrome patient. Their decision to perform the procedure was made in the wake of a tragic event. One of their first patients was afflicted with particularly severe sleep apnea syndrome, and they considered trying the procedure on him, but like Lugaresi and his colleagues they hesitated to take such a drastic step because of suspensions of breathing during sleep. While they were still deliberating, the patient died suddenly from cardiac arrest, only a few days after being examined in the sleep laboratory. This unfortunate event changed their view, so when the next case of sleep apnea syndrome was diagnosed they were ready to operate without delay. Like the others who had performed this procedure before them, Orr and Imes "were left open-mouthed by the dramatic change that took place in the patient and the quality of his sleep."

Meanwhile, in Canada another young physician was having a similar experience. Meir Kryger, who today edits the most comprehensive books on sleep disorders, had been interested in medical research since his student days at McGill University in Montreal. He was particularly intrigued by two subjects, respiratory control and the physiology of the upper airways. He saw his first case of sleep apnea syndrome in 1973: an extremely obese patient who had been considered for a stomach reduction procedure to reduce his weight, and who had been hospitalized with a suspicion of epileptic attacks while asleep. One night, as Kryger visited his patients' rooms, he saw the obese patient choking and suffocating as he slept and decided there and then to examine his sleep. The examination revealed that the patient's difficulties were a result not of epileptic attacks at all, but of prolonged apneas, which caused a dysfunction in heart activity.

Twenty-eight years later, Kryger still does not know how he found the courage to approach the senior physician he was studying under and suggest that he perform a tracheostomy on the obese and sleepy patient; there was very little medical literature at that time dealing with drowsy, obese patients, and the number of tracheostomy procedures performed on them was tiny. For a young, inexperienced intern to suggest such a dramatic procedure solely on the basis of a sleep examination required a great deal of audacity, but to his amazement his superior agreed on the spot. The sleepy, snoring patient received a tracheostomy, and the next night he slept like a babe—in contrast with Kryger himself, who endured several sleepless nights worrying that his decision might, after all, have been the wrong one. The patient, like all his predecessors, had no more "epilepsy" attacks, and he made a complete recovery. Kryger wrote a scientific article—his first ever—describing the "epileptic" case, and it was accepted for publication with no requests for revisions or editing, and not a single comma was changed.

Help from Europe

The first sleep clinic in the United States, named the Sleep Disorders and Research Center, was opened by Bill Dement at Stanford University in 1970, and it constituted a revolution in medical thinking. Until that time, once patients had fallen asleep—even ones who had complained of a sleep disorder—they were considered by doctors to be outside the medical purview. With the opening of the clinic for sleep disorders, for the first time people who had complaints about their sleep were actually examined while they were asleep—and not only that, the examination it-self was conducted by a specialist in sleep disorders. The first patients examined at Stanford were narcoleptics and insomniacs.

As Dement relates in his book *Some Must Watch While Some Must Sleep,* the first two Pickwickian patients were examined at Stanford in 1969. As with all Pickwickians, their breathing was disrupted, but the findings neither aroused any great excitement nor generated a special re-port in the medical literature. To Dement, writing about them seemed superfluous, since Kuhl and Jung, Lugaresi, and Gastaut had already published such reports four years earlier. But the situation at Stanford changed when the laboratory received reinforcements from Europe in the form of Christian Guilleminault, who was to have a decisive influ-ence on the laboratory's activities and on sleep medicine the world over.

Guilleminault was born in Provence, and as a child he never dreamed of becoming either a doctor or sleep researcher; his overriding ambition was to be an explorer and study fascinating cultures. Growing up in an intellectual atmosphere—his father was a newspaper editor and historian, and there were lawyers on his mother's side of the family—he thought his future lay in ethnography, and he saw himself trekking through dense rain forests and discovering new cultures. To this end he began his university studies at seventeen, majoring in the classics, but to his great disappointment he found that he would be unable to embark on his voyages of discovery until he was twenty-five. His mother, more of a pragmatist than her son, convinced him that, as expeditions to far-off lands always needed a doctor, he should study medicine and would thus be able to set off on his travels earlier than expected. Thanks to his mother's suggestion, young Guilleminault found himself studying medicine in Paris.

Following completion of his studies, Guilleminault specialized in neurology and psychiatry at the prestigious La Salpêtrière hospital, home of the greatest French neurologists and psychiatrists. But the adventure bug still gnawed at him, and before completing his internship he decided to enlist in the army. After completing an officer's course near Bordeaux, which helped him to broaden his knowledge of the wonders of French wine, he was assigned as a medical officer to a French expeditionary force bound for North Africa and the Sahara.

After his tour of duty in Africa, Guilleminault returned to Paris to finish his neurology and psychiatry studies, whereupon he had his first encounter with sleep research. To fulfill his psychiatry requirements he decided to write his thesis on the development of intelligence, and in 1962 he went to the University of Geneva to study under Jean Piaget, the high priest of developmental psychology. The Geneva psychiatry department housed one of Europe's first sleep laboratories, under the direction of Miguel Krassoievitch, a native of Argentina. Guilleminault and Krassoievitch, both of whom possessed a Latin temperament and an ardent desire to talk and enjoy themselves deep into the night—so unlike the taciturn Swiss—immediately found common ground. They also shared an interest in sleep. Krassoievitch investigated sleep cycles in senile demented patients, and in 1970 he participated in the first Swiss study of sleep in Pickwickian patients. Guilleminault quickly found himself listening to Piaget's lectures during the day and spending his nights with Krassoievitch in bars and cafés.

Once he finished his doctoral thesis, which applied Piaget's ideas concerning the concept of space in children to dementia patients, Guilleminault returned to Paris, this time as a bona fide doctor. But his experience in Geneva had infected him with an incurable fascination for research, and a short time later he decided on a further turnabout in his life and began doctoral studies in histology at the Paris University of the Sciences. Paris in the late 1960s was an arena for the student revolution, which turned the city's streets into a battleground with the police. Every now and again the police would storm the university lecture halls and laboratories to arrest people they thought had taken part in rioting. To Guilleminault's good fortune, one of his classmates, who happened to be the son of President Georges Pompidou, would warn him of an imminent police swoop on the university.

Guilleminault's first contact with the Stanford sleep laboratory came about by chance. On completing his doctorate, Guilleminault was appointed to a lectureship in neurophysiology at the University of Paris, but since he had a few free months before taking up his new appointment, he decided to spend the time in California, about whose long beaches and pretty girls he had heard a great deal. But all was not tranquil in California, either. Guilleminault arrived in the middle of the student unrest that was sweeping American college campuses as part of the backlash against the war in Vietnam. Nobody, not even at Stanford, had the time or patience for studies or research. Guilleminault, a gregarious young man, quickly acclimatized to Stanford's effervescent environment, and through Steve Henderson, one of the sleep laboratory students whom he helped with histological slides of hamster brains, he soon found himself accepted as a member of Dement's staff at the sleep laboratory.

By the time he returned to France in September 1970, Guilleminault had been truly bitten by the sleep research bug. Although his department head insisted that sleep research was fine for "daydreamers," Guilleminault resigned his appointment and established a sleep laboratory in La Salpêtrière hospital. During the day he functioned as a neurologist, seeing mainly patients with motor dysfunctions, while at night he examined patients in his sleep laboratory, helped by some of his neurophysiology students who worked as volunteer technicians. His efforts, alas, were in vain, for at the end of the year the laboratory's budget ran out and it was threatened with closure. His luck turned again when Bill Dement suggested that he leave Paris and become head of the Stanford sleep unit. And so, in 1972, Christian Guilleminault embarked on his American career—a career that had a decisive effect on sleep medicine in both the United States and the entire world.

The same year, at an American conference on sleep research held at Jackson Hole, Wyoming (and shortly after the Rimini meeting in

Italy), Guilleminault presented the histories of Stanford's first group of patients with sleep apnea syndrome. But the world was still not yet ready to hear about it, and his lecture did not arouse much response. Only one member of the audience was sufficiently interested to ask a question. Guilleminault clearly recalls Peter Hauri, a sleep researcher who, like him, was from Europe, asking it. Hauri, by his own admission, put the question only out of Swiss courtesy.

Thin People Also Stop Breathing in Their Sleep

Until the early 1970s, it was generally accepted that sleep disordered breathing occurred solely in the obese—Pickwickian patients, as they were known in the medical literature. Guilleminault and Dement changed this picture completely when they proved that obesity is not a prerequisite for the existence of these disorders. One of the patients examined at the Stanford sleep laboratory as a result of complaints of difficulty falling asleep and frequent awakenings once he was asleep, was a man of particularly slender build, which on the face of it contradicted the possibility of sleep apneas. In the course of their recordings, Guilleminault and Dement noted that the patient's heartbeat was irregular, and when they went into the bedroom to observe him close up they realized that the source of the irregularity was suspensions of breathing: hundreds of apneas in the course of the night, just like the Pickwickians. Guilleminault and Dement decided that monitoring breathing during sleep should be done for all the patients examined at the Stanford sleep laboratory for any reason at all, not only for Pickwickian patients. This decision was a further milestone in the history of sleep apnea syndrome, for respiratory tests during sleep were not usually part of routine sleep testing. To their great surprise, it quickly became clear that many patients referred for sleep testing due to complaints of tiredness, daytime sleepiness, and even insomnia were in fact suffering from breathing disorders in their sleep—often with no connection at all to their body weight. Like Orr and Imes, Guilleminault and Dement concluded that sleep breathing disorders were by no means exotic, exclusive to a small number of obese people, but common disorders. They were, however, unaware of exactly how common these disorders were.

In 1975 Guilleminault and Dement published an article summarizing their sleep-test findings, including breathing recordings, in 250 patients who had been referred to the Stanford sleep laboratory as a result of complaints of disturbances in their sleep. In 35 of them, the sleep tests showed evidence of breathing disorders, even though not one of the patients had complained of breathing problems during sleep in their pre-test interviews. The article by Guilleminault and his colleagues about these patients was the first to use the term "sleep apnea syndrome," and they also suggested a definition of it in accordance with their laboratory findings. Brief suspensions of breathing during sleep occur in healthy people as well, especially during the falling-asleep process and in REM sleep, but the number of apneas is not usually greater than ten to twenty per night. Sleep apnea syndrome, as defined by Guilleminault and his colleagues, occurs when at least thirty apneas of a minimum duration of ten seconds each are detected during the sleep laboratory examination. To take into account the duration of sleep, which varies from person to person, the definition was later amended to at least five apneas in each hour of sleep.

Although many people still use this definition of the syndrome, as the number of people examined in the sleep laboratory increased it became clear that defining the syndrome solely by the number of apneas was extremely difficult. Using the definition of five apneas in each hour of sleep, it turns out, means that one out of every four men between the ages of forty and sixty suffers from sleep apnea syndrome, as well as almost half the men over sixty. Some researchers therefore use as their criterion ten apneas per hour, or even fifteen or twenty. Others define the syndrome only by a combination of typical complaints, like daytime sleepiness or prolonged tiredness, and the finding of apneas during sleep.

The pioneering study by Guilleminault and his colleagues also produced another noteworthy observation: although the 250 patients tested at the laboratory included an equal number of men and women, of the 35 sleep apnea patients there was only one woman. This was the first evidence that respiratory disorders during sleep are a particular characteristic of men, and it gained much support in the years to come. A further finding, the importance of which became clear only later, was that 16 of the apnea patients suffered from hypertension, and in 3 of them the electrocardiograph recording showed pathological signs. In later years the effect of sleep disorders on the cardiovascular system would become the driving force behind sleep medicine.

The findings disclosed in this important article made the time ripe for an American scientific conference on respiratory disorders in sleep. Ten years after the 1967 Bologna conference, and five years after the one held in Rimini, sleep researchers and specialists in pulmonary physiology gathered at the Kroc Foundation in Santa Inez Valley, California, to examine the accumulated knowledge on respiratory sleep disorders. There is a certain degree of irony in the fact that the conference was held under the aegis of the Kroc Foundation, which was founded by the owner of the giant hamburger chain McDonald's. The Big Mac has contributed perhaps more than anything else to the American fast-food culture, and indirectly to the American obesity epidemic, which in turn is apparently joined at the hip to sleep apnea syndrome.

The Santa Inez conference was attended by all the eminent researchers on respiratory ailments in sleep, including Lugaresi and some of his staff from Bologna, Guilleminault and Dement from Stanford, Daniel Kurtz and Jean Krieger from France, and Elliot Weitzman from New York. Other participants were particularly interested in respiratory functions and control, without any special relationship to sleep, like David Read, a leading Australian pulmonary physician and respiratory physiologist, who later had a major impact on the immediate development of sleep laboratories at the University of Sidney and other places in Australia. But there were also those who began bridging the gap between the two subjects and studying how sleep affects respiratory functions. The most notable of these was Eliot Phillipson of Toronto, who was among the first to renew the pioneering studies of Kleitman, Bulow, and Ingvar on the changes that occur in respiratory control in the transition from wakefulness to sleep.

6

The Dog Dropped Off
and the Experiment Woke Up

We have already seen that the transition between wakefulness and sleep is bound up with variations in respiratory functions. Breathing becomes irregular while a person is falling asleep, with occasional short suspensions, until sleep deepens and stabilizes. Numerous early researchers surmised that this irregularity was caused by a variation in the sensitivity threshold of the cerebral respiratory center to carbon dioxide concentration in the blood, which required a period of adaptation during the transition between wakefulness and sleep. There were those like Kuhl and Jung who assumed that, in people suffering from apneas during the entire course of sleep, the irregular breathing continued beyond the transition period for a reason that was unclear, but very little was known about the physiology of respiratory control during sleep. This picture changed completely by the end of the 1980s thanks mainly to experiments by Eliot Phillipson.

Phillipson completed his medical studies at the University of Alberta, Edmonton, where he specialized in internal medicine. After finishing medical school in 1968, he did postgraduate work at the Cardiovascular Research Institute of the University of California, San Francisco. His research dealt with the functions of the vagus nerve in respiratory control, especially during physical exertion. To this end Phillipson developed a research model that he used, in a controlled experiment, to successfully retard the activity of the vagus nerve in dogs by cooling it, which caused a slowing-down and deepening of the animals' breathing. Following these studies, Phillipson received an academic appointment to the University of Toronto, where he prepared to continue his work on the vagus, a subject he viewed as fertile soil for many years of research. He never imagined that a particularly sleepy dog would bring about a dramatic change in his scientific career.

On a March day in 1973, Phillipson stayed in his laboratory alone to write up the results of an experiment he had just completed, in which he had examined a further aspect of vagus nerve activity. The dog in the experiment stopped running on the treadmill, the recording instruments spewed out data on its respiratory functions, and Phillipson began arranging the data into tables. As he sat at his desk, the dog lay down on the treadmill and fell asleep. A few minutes later, Phillipson went over and found the dog fast asleep, still connected to the instruments measuring its respiratory functions. Nine out of ten researchers would have woken the dog up and disconnected it from the instruments so they could complete their work and go home. But there are researchers whose curiosity is so strong that it does not allow them to miss an opportunity for a further experiment, even an unplanned one. Although Phillipson knew nothing about sleep and was unaware of the existence of respiratory disorders during sleep, he was intrigued by whether vagus activity retardation would affect the sleeping dog to the same degree as it did a wakeful one. So he reactivated the cooling device to retard the sleeping dog's vagus nerve. Initially the variation in the dog's breathing was similar to that observed in a state of wakefulness; the breathing rate slowed and breathing became gradually deeper. But then something else happened, something that Phillipson had never before observed in wakeful dogs: the animal's breathing slowed radically to a rate of three breaths per minute, while at the same time the volume of each inhalation increased to a tremendous one liter, and even more. These variations occurred with no increase in carbon dioxide concentration, which was completely out of line with what the physiology textbooks said about respiratory regulation.

Although this unplanned observation was interesting, Phillipson viewed it as nothing more than an offbeat episode and continued his research on wakeful dogs. Some months later he was invited to the Cardiovascular Research Institute in San Francisco to lecture on his findings on the vagus nerve in respiratory regulation during physical exertion. After the seminar he had a chat in the office of Professor Julius Comroe, the institute's director and one of the greatest researchers on respiratory physiology of his time, whose book *The Lung* was compulsory reading for medical students in the 1960s and '70s. Phillipson told Comroe about his surprising observation with the dog that fell asleep on the treadmill. To his astonishment, Comroe became quite excited. His initial reaction was to ask Phillipson whether it was possible, in his opinion, to investigate respiratory regulation in sleeping dogs. Comroe showed him a copy of the *Bulletin de Physiopathologie Respiratoire* that contained all the papers given at the Rimini conference, and told Phillipson that, according to the articles, disruption of respiratory regulation during sleep was apparently the cause of the Pickwickian syndrome and similar sleep breathing disorders. Comroe went on to say that how the respiratory center works during sleep should be thoroughly investigated to gain a better understanding of the reasons behind sleep disordered breathing. "I warmly recommend," Comroe summed up, "using the research model you have developed to study respiratory regulation during sleep." (The same edition of *Bulletin de Physiopathologie Respiratoire* also played an important role in the career of Colin Sullivan, inventor of the continuous positive air pressure machine, today the most efficacious treatment for sleep apnea syndrome.)

Back home in Toronto, Phillipson borrowed some electrophysiological recording instruments from hospital colleagues and set up a laboratory to investigate the respiratory functions of sleeping dogs—a move that surprised many of his friends, who found it hard to understand why he would abandon a research subject as promising as the influence of the vagus nerve on respiratory functions for one as marginal as respiratory regulation in sleep. But results were not long in coming, and Phillipson's change of research direction was a smart one. In early 1975, at a conference of the American Physiological Society, he presented the results of his first study on respiratory regulation in sleep, and in July 1977 his first scientific article on the subject was published. He also attended the Santa Inez conference of 1977, and it is not surprising that his opening sentence there was: "It will be impossible to discover the mechanism and causes of breathing disorders during sleep, and of sleep apnea, without understanding the normal functioning of the regulatory mechanisms of breathing during sleep." In this lecture he summarized his main findings of the previous two years, which shed new light on the regulation of breathing during sleep.

The "Automatic Pilot" in Sleep

Phillipson conducted all his experiments on dogs that had been trained to sleep in the laboratory while connected to the recording instruments. The measurements were usually performed in the afternoon, some two hours after the dogs had been fed, so they would fall asleep more easily. As with all mammals, the sleep of dogs is composed of two types. During the first type, which is characterized by slow, regular brain waves, the muscles are lax and pulse rate, blood pressure, and breathing are regular and moderate. The second type of sleep is characterized by rapid and disorganized brain waves, disappearance of muscle tone, rapid eye movements similar to those during wakefulness, muscle spasms, and intensive activity of the autonomic nervous system manifested by frequent variations in pulse rate, breathing, and blood pressure. In humans this sleep stage is characterized by dreaming. The first type, with its slow, regular brain waves, is called non-REM sleep; the second type, with its rapid eye movements, is known as REM sleep.

In his first series of experiments, Phillipson examined the respiratory response to variations in carbon dioxide levels in both sleep stages. As noted earlier, the carbon dioxide level is the most important stimulus for activation of the respiratory center in the brain stem. Phillipson found that in non-REM sleep, a rise in the carbon dioxide concentration caused a gradual increase in breathing rate and volume until the dog woke up. In REM sleep the reaction was completely different. The breathing pattern in REM sleep, which is usually unstable and may vary from one moment to the next from slow to rapid and vice versa, is almost unaffected by variations in carbon dioxide level. Despite the increase in the concentration of the gas being identical to that in non-REM sleep, the variations in breathing rate and volume in REM sleep were small and insignificant. Similar differences between the two types of sleep were also found regarding the effect of variations in the blood oxygen saturation level. In non-REM sleep, the reaction to a drop in the blood oxygen saturation level was immediate, while in REM sleep a relatively long time elapsed before the respiratory center reacted by increasing the breathing rate. As a result, the blood oxygen saturation level that caused awakening from REM sleep was much lower than in non-REM sleep.

Phillipson concluded that different regulatory mechanisms control breathing in non-REM and REM sleep. In non-REM sleep, breathing is under the control of the automatic, or metabolic, breathing mechanism located in the brain stem's respiratory center, which acts as an "automatic pilot." It receives information from many and varied sources, such as the chemical sensors located in the brain stem that are sensitive to blood gas levels, the mechanical sensors in the lung walls that track the degree of lung tension, and the sensors that are sensitive to airflow in the upper airways; depending on the sum total of information that flows into it, the respiratory center varies the breathing rate and volume. For example, when the respiratory center receives signals during non-REM sleep informing it of an increase in the carbon dioxide level, or of a drop in the blood oxygen level, it immediately acts to increase breathing rate and intensity. When it receives information on oxygen levels that are too high or carbon dioxide levels that are too low, the center acts to reduce breathing rate and depth, even to the point of cessation.

Breathing in REM sleep, by contrast, is controlled not by the automatic system but by the "voluntary" respiratory center located in the frontal lobe of the cerebrum. This is the regulatory center that enables us to slow down or accelerate our breathing as we wish, or to stop it for short periods. It takes over especially during active states, such as while we talk, laugh, cry, or swallow, and its action is reduced during states of inactivity. This center is less sensitive to stimuli from the respiratory system than the respiratory centers in the brain stem, and so in REM sleep there is a reduced reaction both to variations in blood gas levels and to other respiratory stimuli from the lungs, the thoracic muscles, or the flow and pressure sensors in the uppper airways. The reason that breathing during REM sleep is irregular is connected to the special characteristics of this type of sleep. The irregular breathing intensifies with the appearance of the rapid eye movements characteristic of REM sleep, which indicates that the variations in breathing are only a part of a general neural activity pattern that goes into action during REM sleep.

The action of the respiratory system during sleep therefore can be likened to that of the automatic pilot in an airplane. In the absence of a guiding human hand, the working of the automatic pilot relies on a constant flow of information from the aircraft's various systems. In contrast, in REM sleep the automatic pilot is disconnected from these systems and acts in accordance with a preset program, which receives data on the aircraft's altitude, airspeed, and course. Yet the flight is not steady, and the automatic pilot finds it difficult to absorb information from the aircraft's systems and correct the flight data accordingly, except in situations of extreme danger.

The implications of Phillipson's findings for sleep apnea syndrome were several. First, his conclusions focused attention on the importance of the automatic mechanism that regulates breathing during sleep. Every malfunction in the activity of the metabolic mechanism is liable to cause suspension of breathing. It is possible, Phillipson claims, that during sleep there is a reduction in the information flow from the various sensors to the respiratory center, and this is liable to cause malfunction in respiratory functions. Another possibility is a defect in the nerve cells of the brain's respiratory center that are unable to process the information reaching them in a normal fashion. This defect will not cause suspensions of breathing during wakefulness, because the wakefulness mechanisms located close to the respiratory center in the brain stem ensure that respiratory activity continues as usual. According to Phillipson, the wakefulness mechanism also ensures the renewal of breathing during sleep. The increased concentration of carbon dioxide and the reduced level of oxygen in the blood cause activation of the wakefulness mechanism, and also the renewal of breathing. In other words, this is clearly a defense mechanism, and if it were not activated sleep apnea would cause people to suffocate in their sleep.

The findings indicating that respiratory regulation in REM sleep is controlled by a separate mechanism raised the possibility that apneas during this sleep stage are connected to a malfunction of the voluntary control mechanisms, and not to a malfunction of the metabolic mechanism. This can explain why there are those who experience apneas only during REM sleep, not during non-REM sleep, and others who have apneas only during non-REM sleep, and why, when the apneas appear in both types of sleep, they are more prolonged and severe during REM sleep. As noted earlier, during REM sleep the respiratory mechanisms react extremely slowly to variations in blood gas levels and other stimuli originating in breathing, so a relatively long time elapses until the wakefulness mechanism goes into action and renews breathing.

An additional reason why apneas during REM sleep last longer than in non-REM sleep is that in REM sleep there is a significant reduction in muscle tonus, which resembles a state of muscular paralysis. This reduction causes a further narrowing of the airways and also a reduced respiratory reaction at the conclusion of the apnea.

Although the majority of Phillipson's findings withstood the test of time, Comroe's hypothesis that an understanding of the activity of the respiratory mechanisms during sleep would clarify the causes of sleep apnea syndrome remained unfulfilled.

Airway Collapse: An Active or Passive Episode?

Another topic widely discussed at Santa Inez, and which in recent years has become a central research subject of sleep apnea syndrome, is where the upper airway blockage actually occurs, and why. At the conference, researchers presented the first attempts to identify the location of the blockage in an effort to understand the reasons behind it, including a peep into the pharynx of a male who suffered from sleep apnea. Elliot Weitzman, a medical school classmate of Dement's who, like Dement, gained prominence as one of America's leading sleep researchers, set up one of the first sleep disorder clinics in the United States at the Montefiore Medical Center in the Bronx, New York. At the Santa Inez conference, Weitzman and his colleagues presented one of the first experiments to precisely pinpoint the blockage site in the airways of sleep apnea syndrome patients. They used a fluoroscopy, which is a dynamic X-ray viewing method that enabled them to follow what was taking place at various locations in the sleep apnea patient's airways during the different stages of his suspensions of breathing. Later endoscopy, which utilizes optic fibers inserted through the nostrils down the throat, was used for the same purpose. As a result of their excessive sleepiness, sleep apnea patients can fall asleep at any time and under any conditions, so Weitzman and his colleagues had no difficulty in performing this examination while their patient was asleep.

The fluoroscopy showed that the cause of the blockage was a collapse of the side walls of the pharynx and a backward movement of the base of the tongue. This "landslide" always occurred at the end of exhalation and before the next inhalation, and as the pharynx was blocked, the movements of the diaphragm and thoracic muscles "sucked" the soft tissues and the tongue into the pharynx, thus creating negative pressure in the thorax and causing the total blockage of the pharynx until the moment of awakening, when the airways opened and breathing was renewed.

The observations of Weitzman and his colleagues confirmed Gerardy's first reports from 1960 on the backward movement of the tongue during apneas. At the same conference, Ron Harper of Los Angeles complemented Weitzman's observations by reporting that during an apnea there is a reduction in the intensity of the tongue muscles' electrical activity, which facilitates the tongue's backward movement.

But what is the cause of the laxity of the muscles of the pharynx walls and the oral cavity, and the weakness of the lingual muscles at the beginning of inhalation? And why does it occur only in some people and not all of us?

Following Weitzman's lecture there was a lively discussion on the video films he presented. Weitzman claimed that the sleep films showed that the muscles in the oropharynx area, which are smooth muscles—

that is, muscles that are not under voluntary control—were actively contracted during the apnea. In other words, because of a malfunction in the
respiratory center's activity, the muscles receive an erroneous command
from the brain and instead of dilating they constrict and the airways
close. Others rejected this notion and fervently argued that the airway
walls collapse passively only because of the negative pressure created in
the thorax during inhalation. Furthermore, Guilleminault and his Stanford colleagues also used endoscopic photography during sleep and
reached a completely contradictory conclusion. They claimed that this
was not an active blockage of the airways, but rather a passive collapse of
the pharynx walls.

There were also those who raised another possibility: a timing malfunction in the action of the muscles that widen the pharynx and not a
reduction of its force. As during normal breathing the upper airway muscles contract with precise timing, thus ensuring the opening of the airways, then if even a single muscle contracts too early the delicate structure is liable to collapse and cause a blockage of the airways.

The reverberations from the Santa Inez discussion continued to
echo for a long time in the professional literature. Although today there
is a consensus that airway collapse is not caused by an active contraction
of the smooth muscles in the pharynx walls, the reasons for the collapse
are still unknown. Unfortunately, Elliot Weitzman, who had such a bril-
liant future in sleep research, died of cancer in 1984.

What Causes Upper Airway Collapse?

The upper airways of sleep apnea patients became a scientific challenge
for numerous research groups throughout the world. All of them probed
the oral cavity with fine needles and sensitive electrodes for measuring
the electrical activity of the smooth muscles in order to investigate how
they react to pressure variations during sleep.

The opening of the upper airways is dependent on the normal action of the muscles that widen the airways. These muscles, which cover
the area of the oral cavity and pharynx like a wide ring, prevent the walls

from adhering to one another when negative pressure is created in the thorax during inhalation and are subordinate to two types of mechanism. One type of muscle is automatically activated by the respiratory mechanism and its action is coordinated with respiratory movement, so that the muscles widen the airways with each inhalation. In contrast, tonus in the second type of muscle is constant and the muscles are activated by reflexes. The source of stimulus for the activation of the reflex is in the sensitive sensors for airflow and pressure, located in the pharynx walls and the oral cavity. The moment that air flows over them, or when they sense a change of pressure resulting from the expansion of the thorax, they signal the brain's respiratory center, which in response commands the activation of the muscles, thus widening the airways. In this way the two mechanisms ensure the widening of the upper airways with each breath taken.

During sleep, when the effect of stimuli from the wakefulness center diminishes, the information received from the airflow and pressure sensors in the airways becomes more important, and any disruption of the information flow may cause a disruption in the respiratory center's activity. In 1982, Eliot Phillipson spent a sabbatical at the Technion Sleep Laboratory in Haifa. This was a golden opportunity for us to hear first-hand about respiratory functions from one of the world's leading researchers of this subject, and with him we planned a number of joint studies. In one of these experiments we examined the importance of the air sensors in the nose and pharynx with regard to respiratory functions during sleep. To this end we paralyzed the sensors using a lidocaine spray, a local anesthetic whose effects last for a few hours. This was done to healthy subjects who were not afflicted with any kind of sleep disorder, a few minutes before they went to sleep in the laboratory.

On examination of the first volunteer we could already see how vital the normal function of the sensors is to the regularity of breathing during sleep. A few minutes after the subject fell asleep, he stopped breathing for a period of fifty seconds. The apnea was central—that is, the brain's respiratory center ceased its activity, as we could learn from the fact that the airflow ceased and the respiratory muscles or the diaphragm did not move at all. We had never seen such a prolonged apnea in healthy subjects at the onset of sleep. Additional apneas appeared later, with their number gradually diminishing as the effect of the anesthetic decreased. All the subjects who participated in the experiment experienced apneas in the first hour or two of their sleep as a result of anesthetizing the nose and pharynx. On the other hand, the anesthetic had no effect on any of the subjects' breathing during wakefulness. Yet despite these dramatic findings we did not continue with the study of the sensors' functioning during sleep. The Lebanon War of 1982, which broke out a short time after Phillipson came to Haifa, wrecked all the sleep laboratory's plans for that year.

A study of the necessity of the nose's air sensors for normal breathing during sleep was also one of the first research projects undertaken by David White, head of the Harvard Sleep Research Laboratory and clinical director of the Sleep HealthCenters in Boston. White joined the circle of sleep researchers after completing his medical studies at Emory University in Georgia and specializing in pulmonary medicine at the National Jewish Medical and Research Center in Denver. White and his colleagues showed that local anesthetization of the nostrils caused a fourfold increase in the number of apneas in healthy subjects.

White's research group is currently engaged in the study of muscle activity in the upper airways with the aim of solving the riddle of their failure in sleep apnea patients. By introducing tiny electrodes into a group of muscles in the upper airways, White succeeded in recording their electrical activity during sleep and wakefulness, in both healthy subjects and sleep apnea patients. To a certain extent, his first findings were paradoxical: during wakefulness, the activity of muscles expanding the airways was more vigorous in sleep apnea patients than in the healthy subjects. White's explanation for this was that the airways of sleep apnea patients are narrower than those of healthy people, and so they need increased muscle activity to compensate for it and ensure a normal airflow. The sleep apnea patients manage to overcome the narrowing of their airways only during wakefulness, however. The increased activity of the smooth muscles disappears during sleep, while the muscle activity of healthy subjects is heightened.

Today, after devoting twenty years to studying the functioning of the upper airways, White is far wiser about the possible causes of sleep apnea. He does not believe that the "landslide" in the airways during sleep can be explained by the failure of a single mechanism. In his view, it is quite possible that various mechanisms are involved in the syndrome—some linked to an interruption in the activity of the expanding muscles, and others connected with the respiratory regulating mechanisms during sleep.

The Snoring Continuum

The upper airways, from the nose to the trachea, are a complex, delicate system under the strict supervision of the respiratory center in the brain. The sensors located along its length provide the control center in the brain with continuous reports on the airflow and pressure situation throughout the "pipeline." This information is processed and, in a flash, commands are transmitted to the smooth muscles in the airway walls to change their degree of contraction.

In healthy people without sleep or breathing disorders, too, the changes in the airways cause a slight disruption of the function of the respiratory center—a change of posture, such as moving from a sitting to a standing position, for example, or the change in the brain's condition from wakefulness to sleep. Even astronauts, who undergo the strictest medical examinations, experience mild breathing disorders during sleep. In a study of the sleep of five astronauts conducted by a group of researchers from the University of California at San Diego and Harvard University, in conjunction with NASA, it was found that before liftoff into space, the astronauts experienced 8.3 full or partial apneas in an average hour and that they snored for 16 percent of their sleep time. The majority of these apneas ended with a brief awakening. One of the five astronauts who participated in the study experienced 22 such episodes in an hour! In addition to the recordings conducted before the launch, four sleep recordings were conducted on all the astronauts while they were in space and afterward. The recordings conducted in space under conditions of weightlessness were extremely surprising. In all the subjects there was a sharp drop in the number of full and partial apneas, from 8.3 to 3.4 per hour, and with them the number of awakenings was reduced. Not only that, but snoring disappeared completely. The sleep recordings conducted after their return to Earth showed that the situation was as before: the astronauts were snoring again and the number of respiratory episodes rose to 9.5 per hour.

The researchers concluded that sleep in an environment without the force of gravity made a significant contribution to breathing because of the drop in resistance to airflow. Freedom from the force of gravity enables astronauts to sleep either standing or lying down, as long as they are belted in position and cannot float around the capsule. Under such conditions there is no collapse of the soft tissues in the area of the pharynx and oral cavity, which ensures normal airflow as during wakefulness. In recent years it has become clear that only the slightest of variations in the pressure created in the airways may sometimes cause significant sleep disorders, even without a partial collapse in the airways.

In 1993, Guilleminault and his colleagues proposed the term "upper airway resistance syndrome" to describe the problem experienced by a group of patients who had been examined in their sleep laboratory for complaints of excessive drowsiness and chronic fatigue with no apparent reason. These people awakened from their sleep on numerous occasions for a period of five to ten seconds. The immediate reason for these awakenings was variations in the negative pressure in the thorax and a slight, almost undetectable reduction in airflow. The raised negative pressure caused activation of the wakefulness mechanisms in the brain and interruption of the normal course of sleep. The recurring interruption of sleep is apparently the cause of the chronic fatigue that afflicts people with the syndrome. In contrast to sleep apnea syndrome, which can be easily diagnosed by recording respiratory function during sleep, diagnosing upper airway resistance syndrome is no simple matter. Recording airflow and thoracic contractions does not contribute to the diagnosis, because the variations in breathing from this syndrome are so slight that their detection is difficult. The only way to diagnose the syndrome is by monitoring pressure variations in the thorax during sleep, and this is done by introducing a sensor connected to a sphygmoma-

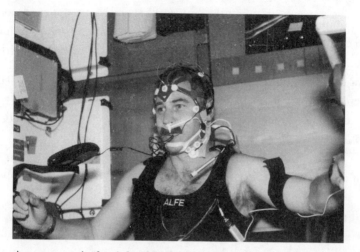

An astronaut in the *Columbia* space shuttle ready for a sleep study

nometer into the esophagus. It is determined that the patient is encountering the syndrome when the brief awakenings appear close to the rise in negative pressure in the thorax. This syndrome—which may not even be associated with snoring—is apparently the most simple form of sleep disordered breathing. The reason for the phenomenon is not clear, but the fact that the majority of people in whom upper airway resistance was found have a narrowing of the airways indicates that the cause is linked to a minor airflow disruption due to the structure of the airways.

Elio Lugaresi was the first to raise the possibility of a snoring continuum, with light snorers who show no evidence of sleep disordered breathing at one end, and at the other those whose stentorian snoring is recurrently interrupted by prolonged apneas and who endure a significant drop in their blood oxygen and a rise in blood carbon dioxide. In the most severe cases, the blood oxygen level is low and carbon dioxide level high even during the day.

Between the two ends of the scale are the less severe breathing disorders, such as the upper airway resistance described by Guilleminault, or breathing disorders during sleep that are manifested by a partial blockage of the airways. It is not clear at this stage, however, how the non-snoring patients with increased upper airway resistance fit into this continuum. Although the various breathing disorders differ in number and duration in their degree of blood oxygen reduction and the physical effort that accompanies renewal of breathing, they all have a common denominator—the recurring interruption of the continuous course of sleep. When sleep is interrupted numerous times, even for periods not exceeding five to ten seconds, it is in no way refreshing, and as a result daytime wakefulness is low and functioning is impaired.

Many studies attempted to determine whether a person who was found to be only a snorer might develop full-blown sleep apnea after a few years. The results are not uniform and in some cases are even contradictory. In the majority of subjects who were examined every few years, no dramatic variations were found in respiratory function during sleep, unless there was a radical variation in the person's weight or in the structure of the upper airways. When we examined forty sleep apnea patients in the sleep laboratory five years after their first examination, we found no great change in the severity of their respiratory disorders. The average number of apneas in the first examination was twenty-seven per hour, compared with twenty-eight in the second. We also did not find any variation in these patients' body weight or in their complaints. A young man in his thirties with upper airway resistance syndrome is not at high risk of contracting severe sleep apnea syndrome, on condition that he watches his weight and does not overindulge in alcoholic beverages before going to sleep. It is almost certain that in those who reported loud snoring before the appearance of apneas, the situation worsened with the years, and particularly with changes in body weight.

Because there are quite a few apneas even in the sleep of healthy people, and because they do not bring other sleep disorders in their wake, there is a need for a clear definition of the borders separating the normal from the pathological. It is currently agreed that a diagnosis of sleep apnea syndrome should require full or partial apneas, or even a slight increase in upper airway resistance, in addition to complaints of excessive fatigue or drowsiness. However, I shall return to the question of the definition of sleep apnea syndrome later, when we discuss the cardiovascular consequences of the syndrome.

7

From an Exotic Syndrome
to a Public Health Issue

The reports published in scientific journals in the 1970s about patients suffocating in their sleep, and stating that the only way to diagnose them was by means of examination during sleep, did nothing to change the medical world's attitude toward the subject of sleep. The excitement of sleep researchers did not infect their colleagues, and hospital administrations did not hasten to establish laboratories for the diagnosis of sleep disorders. In many countries there was no sleep medicine at all, and worldwide it was the occupation of only a few hundred sleep researchers. Most of them were engaged in basic sleep research and did not show any particular interest in sleep disorders. Before sleep medicine could become fully accepted, it first had to establish that sleep breathing disorders were not mere medical anecdotes but a common occurrence affecting large numbers of people. Finding out the prevalence of the syndrome in the general population required epidemiological research—the investigation of the incidence and prevalence of disease in large populations, as well as the causes.

A properly conducted epidemiological study is no easy task. Drawing conclusions about the entire population requires a sufficiently large representative sample. A decision has to be made on the method

79

to be used for gathering the information, whether by interviews, questionnaires, or sleep examinations. Data must be gathered accurately and reliably, and it is necessary to set clear criteria for defining "sick" and "healthy" people.

Snoring in San Marino

Epidemiological studies are sometimes the result of the clinical intuition of an astute physician, one who has detected a connection between symptoms and a particular illness in a small number of cases. This was the case with the first epidemiological study on sleep disordered breathing. Immediately after the first sleep examinations of Pickwickian patients in Bologna, Lugaresi and his colleagues noted that in many cases complaints of loud snoring preceded other symptoms, such as tiredness, sleepiness, or hypertension, by several years. This observation, which led Lugaresi to hypothesize the continuum of snoring, also led to the first epidemiological study on sleep disorders and snoring. In 1976, a dedicated and industrious medical student interviewed 5,713 of the 20,000 adult inhabitants of the Republic of San Marino in eastern Italy.

San Marino was ideal for this kind of study. Its residents enjoy free medical insurance, and health services in the tiny country, which covers only sixty square kilometers, are organized in an exemplary fashion. The fact that Lugaresi was born only thirty kilometers from San Marino and was personally acquainted with all its doctors and—even more important—with all its local politicians undoubtedly contributed to the selection of this location for the study. Personal interviews with the residents of San Marino included questions about the quality of their sleep, their use of sleep medication, and the nature and loudness of their snoring, as well as questions on medical history and general health.

The findings revealed that snoring is very common. About 45 percent of those interviewed reported that they snored occasionally, and 25 percent that they snored every day. The incidence of snoring increased with age and was higher among men than women; it was also higher among the obese than those of normal weight. At age forty, 30 percent of men and 20 percent of women snored regularly; for those over sixty these figures rose to 50 percent for men and 40 percent for women.

But the most impressive findings pertained to the connection between snoring and hypertension. People who snored every night—men and women, thin and obese, young and old—all had higher blood pressure than those who did not snore at all. These differences were particularly prominent among thin people younger than fifty. The San Marino study was the first to show that sleep disordered breathing was not an exotic occurrence but highly common, especially among adults. Although it was impossible to discern how many of the snorers experienced apneas during sleep, the connection between snoring and apnea indicated that a large proportion of the adult population was living with it.

Countries like Finland, Sweden, and Denmark are also ideal for epidemiological studies, for two main reasons: first, meticulous medical records are maintained for each and every resident, and, second, Scandinavians are known for their willingness to fill out medical questionnaires that they receive by mail. One of the most notable Scandinavian epidemiological studies was conducted on twins in Finland in 1975. It investigated the significance of genetic factors, compared with environmental ones, in the development of various diseases. Under the direction of Markku Koskenvuo from the University of Turkku, researchers distributed questionnaires to twenty thousand pairs of identical and fraternal twins, who were asked to provide detailed information on their health, eating and drinking habits, other life routines, and medical histories. Researchers continue to send the twins additional questionnaires every few years to keep abreast of any changes.

Markku Partinen, who studied medicine at the University of Montpellier in France, was the first sleep researcher in Finland. Since he was familiar with Lugaresi and his research and had even studied epidemiology, he persuaded the twin study's medical committee to include questions about snoring and sleep disorders in the questionnaires distributed in 1981. Since then, the Finnish twins have provided an unfailing source of information on sleep disorders, one that has yielded several scientific publications. It was discovered, for instance, that genetic factors influence the duration and quality of sleep more than environmen-

tal ones, that one in every thirty thousand Finns is afflicted with narcolepsy, and that one in every ten grinds his or her teeth during sleep. Of
particular interest were the findings on the Finnish twins' snoring habits
and the connection between snoring and heart conditions. First, perhaps to the relief of the residents of San Marino, people in the cold countries of the north also snore. Nine percent of men and 4 percent of women
between forty and fifty-nine reported that they snored every night; 20
percent snored frequently, 60 percent snored occasionally, and only 10
percent did not snore at all. In other words, about a quarter of all Finnish
twins snored frequently or even more often. Like the findings of Lugaresi
and his colleagues, this study showed that snoring is more prevalent
among obese people and smokers. It also revealed that twice as many
men and women who snored regularly suffered from hypertension than
men and women who did not snore at all. The connection between snoring and hypertension was particularly prominent in men and women
under fifty and was detected in both thin and obese people.

Three years later, when questionnaires were again sent to the twins,
it transpired that those who had previously reported that they always
snored or snored frequently ran twice the risk of contracting coronary
artery disease as those who snored occasionally or not at all. This connection was not contingent on body weight, hypertension, smoking, or
alcohol intake.

The San Marino findings, as well as those from Finland, indicated
that one in every four adults attests to snoring frequently at least. But because snoring is only one of the symptoms of sleep apnea syndrome and
does not necessarily indicate suspension of breathing during sleep, a further study was required to address the question of how many of the snorers actually suffer from sleep apnea.

Is the Worker's Sleep Indeed Sweet?

At the Technion Sleep Laboratory toward the end of the 1970s, we
began examining people who complained of sleep-related problems.
Like everyone else, we were convinced at the time that we would be deal-

ing only with insomnia or narcolepsy, and did not anticipate that most people who came to us for consultation would complain of chronic tiredness and sleepiness. Scientific literature did not discuss this type of complaint until the 1980s, and studies on the prevalence of sleep disorders did not address complaints of prolonged tiredness or excessive sleepiness. We therefore undertook a planned study to investigate the prevalence of these complaints in the general population in Israel. But how could the prevalence of complaints that are apparently so trivial be studied accurately? It sometimes seemed that statements like "I'm always tired" or "I want to sleep all the time" were the trademark of every middle-aged man. Should it therefore be determined that all men suffer from chronic tiredness? To obtain data that did not express a state of mind but indicated an actual disorder, we approached a large medical institute that specialized in periodic medical examinations of workers. The examinations included a detailed health questionnaire, followed by an interview with the institute physician. Since the patient knew that upon completion of the questionnaire the physician would interview him painstakingly, it could be confidently assumed that people who stated that they sleep "too much" actually meant it.

When we analyzed the answers of about fifteen thousand respondents, we discovered that 4 percent of them complained of chronic tiredness and that they sleep "too much." Although this figure was much smaller than the 18 percent who complained of difficulties in falling asleep or waking up frequently, it was far higher than anything previously reported in medical literature. Unlike complaints of insomnia, however, which were more prevalent among women than men and whose incidence increased with age, the complaints of tiredness and excessive sleeping were more prevalent among men and were similar in all age groups.

These findings corroborated our impression that large numbers of people complain of prolonged tiredness and sleeping too much, but do not normally get attention. Indeed, it is very easy to disregard complaints considered so trivial. Many recounted that when they complained to their family doctor about their propensity to fall asleep in various situations during the day, their doctor's response was placatory and even dismissive: "You're lucky to be able to sleep well, I wish I could." Some reported that their doctor recommended a long vacation to overcome cumulative tiredness. Their argument that the propensity to fall asleep during the day was exacerbated on vacations was usually disregarded.

To examine the reasons for complaints of tiredness and sleepiness, we conducted a further study of more than fifteen hundred industrial workers. They were interviewed in great detail about sleeping habits, disturbances during night sleep, disruptions in levels of attentiveness during the day, health condition, use of medication, satisfaction with the workplace, and more. Based on their responses, about one hundred of the workers were invited to come for sleep examinations at the laboratory, among them some who complained about disturbances in their sleep and their level of attentiveness, and others who did not complain of problems of this kind. The sleep laboratory test findings clearly showed that the primary reason for complaints about tiredness and excessive sleepiness during the day was sleep disordered breathing. Half the workers who complained about excessive sleeping and were tested in the laboratory experienced more than ten apneas per hour during sleep. Based on statistical analysis of the findings, at least one in every hundred men in Israel over age twenty-one, and four in every hundred men over forty, are afflicted with sleep apnea syndrome. When we compared the workers who had sleep breathing disorders with their counterparts, we discovered several differences. Sleep disordered breathing was closely connected to hypertension, headaches on waking up in the morning, loud and disturbing snoring, and excessive daytime sleepiness—all of which are characteristic of people with sleep apnea syndrome.

When I first presented our findings at an international conference of sleep researchers, one prominent American researcher commented with a hint of sarcasm, "It would appear that breathing disorders during sleep are particularly prevalent in the Middle East." He did not believe that possibly 4 percent of people aged forty to sixty suffer from sleep disordered breathing. It quickly transpired that the Middle East is not the exception. Similar studies conducted in different parts of the world at the time revealed similar findings. In Italy, Scandinavia, Germany, and the United States, between 1 and 4 percent of the total adult population was found to have sleep apnea syndrome. The variations in findings between

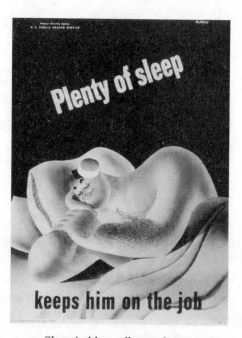

Sleep in blue collar workers—
an educational poster distributed
by the U.S. Public Health Service
in 1942 on the importance of sleep

the different studies were negligible and could be explained by such factors as whether the study included people who were apparently healthy or sick, or young or old; what definition of the syndrome was used, such as five apneas or ten apneas per hour; and whether, in addition to the laboratory findings, complaints of tiredness and sleepiness were also taken into account. All the studies, however, revealed a higher prevalence of the syndrome among men than among women and in obese people than in the thin, and that it tends to increase with age, especially in women.

In the spring of 1982, Lugaresi and his colleagues organized a conference on the epidemiology of sleep disorders in Milano Maritima, a picturesque resort on the Adriatic coast. Most of the researchers actively working on epidemiological studies attended the conference. Markku Partinen reported on the initial findings of the Finnish twin study, Guilleminault and Dement from Stanford reported on sleep disorders in northern California, Daniel Kripke reported on the prevalence of sleep breathing disorders in retirement homes in San Diego, Richard Coleman summarized the accumulated experience of diagnosing sleep disorders in sleep laboratories throughout the United States, Lugaresi and his colleagues reported on the San Marino findings, and I reported on the findings of the study of industrial workers from Haifa.

Although I have attended dozens of scientific conferences throughout the world since the one in Milano Maritima, this one left an indelible impression, and not only because of the quality of the Italian cuisine we enjoyed every evening. It was clearly stated for the first time that sleep disorders, and especially breathing disorders during sleep, are more widely prevalent in the general population than familiar diseases that have been known for many years, such as asthma, Parkinson's disease, or epilepsy. In retrospect, I believe that at the time even the conference participants themselves did not fully appreciate the significance of the findings for public health, on one hand, and the future of sleep medicine on the other. One of the conference highlights was a tourist excursion to San Marino, the only country in the world with a documented intensity of snoring in one-fourth of its residents. At the reception held in our honor, it was evident that Lugaresi, had he so desired, could have easily been elected prime minister.

The Sleep of Civil Service Workers in Wisconsin

Although the reports on snoring habits and sleep apnea syndrome appeared in reputable scientific publications, being published in one of the most prestigious medical journals, such as the *New England Journal of Medicine, The Lancet,* or the *British Medical Journal,* was necessary to "legitimize" the findings. A number of years later such an endorsement did indeed occur, and it changed everything.

There is a long-standing tradition of productive research on respiratory control at the University of Wisconsin. Jerome Dempsey, Hubert Forster, and Gerald Bisgard, known in the field as the Wisconsin Group, researched the activity of chemical sensors in the brain stem and the mechanisms for tolerance to hypoxia. In 1986, Dempsey approached Terry Young, a talented epidemiologist from the department of preventive medicine at the University of Wisconsin, who was researching cancer risk factors, with a proposition to participate in an extensive study financed by the National Institutes of Health on the prevalence of sleep disordered breathing in the general population. At the time, Young knew very little about sleep and was unaware of the existence of sleep breathing disorders. Before deciding to accept Dempsey's proposition, she reviewed the scientific literature on the subject and discovered that almost nothing was being done about the matter in the United States. The only articles she came across were from faraway places like Israel, Italy, and Scandinavia. The proposition therefore posed a great challenge for her. Rather than being one of many people researching cancer risk factors, she now had an opportunity to pioneer a completely new field in which no American epidemiologist had been involved thus far. From the moment she reached a decision, Young attests, "not a single day went by that I did not think about breathing disorders during sleep, and the subject became a central part of my life."

The most important prerequisite for a successful epidemiological study is selection of a sample that will accurately represent the population. It is also advisable to select a sample that will enable follow-up of the participants over a number of years. There are several methods of selecting a representative sample, one of which is random selection of names from a telephone directory and calling the people to solicit their participation in the study. The composition of this type of sample is contingent on people answering the telephone, so the likelihood that people who do not work will fall into the sample is relatively high and it can therefore lean toward overrepresentation of the sick or disabled. To avoid this type of bias and to ensure that all participants in the study were healthy, Young selected a sample of civil service workers in Wisconsin. An added advantage to selecting civil service workers is that their personal details are available to anyone. The researchers conducting the study had access to the names of all State of Wisconsin employees, from which they selected about three thousand people between ages thirty and sixty. Young and her team approached each worker who came up in the sample with a personal letter, accompanied by information on sleep and its significance. The personal approach and exposure of the study in the media have so far led to fifteen hundred of the civil service workers agreeing to sleep in the University of Wisconsin's sleep laboratory in the interest of science. To ensure the participants' agreement to undergo further laboratory examinations in the course of the study, the research team has endeavored to make the laboratory examination as enjoyable an experience as possible.

In the first of many studies on the prevalence of sleep apnea syndrome, 602 people were examined overnight at the sleep laboratory, of whom 355 were defined as "snorers" and 247 as "non-snorers." The definition of sleep apnea syndrome was based on the combination of two criteria: five full or partial apneas per hour, or approximately thirty episodes in the course of an entire night, in addition to subjective complaints of sleepiness during the day.

The study's findings were quite dramatic. One in every four men and one in every ten women had at least five breathing disruptions in one hour of sleep; 15 percent of the men and 5 percent of the women experienced at least ten episodes per hour; and 9 percent of the men and 4 percent of the women had at least fifteen per hour. These findings indicated that sleep disordered breathing is highly prevalent. When complaints of daytime sleepiness were taken into account, it was determined that 2 percent of the women and 4 percent of the men between thirty and sixty had sleep apnea syndrome, similar to the reports in Scandinavia, Italy, Germany, and Israel. (When only laboratory findings are taken into account, disregarding subjective complaints, the syndrome's prevalence is at least twice as great.) Unlike previous findings that left almost no impression on the medical community, however, the influence of Young and her research partners' findings was immense. Almost overnight, sleep apnea syndrome became a central issue in public medicine. There were two main reasons for this: first, contrary to previous studies conducted by sleep researchers, who used epidemiologists to analyze the findings, this was the first time an epidemiologist actively led a sleep study that was meticulously conducted in accordance with rules of epidemiological research. Second, the findings were published in the *New England Journal of Medicine,* the most respected medical journal and the one more widely read than any other. The journal's editors even devoted a special editorial written by Eliot Phillipson to the study conducted by Young and her colleagues. The title of the editorial was "Sleep Apnea Syndrome: A Major Public Health Problem."

The paper by Terry Young and her colleagues, published in 1993, has so far been quoted thousands of times and has become a milestone in the history of sleep apnea syndrome.

8

Risk Factors for Sleep Apnea

On long transatlantic flights, I make a point of walking several times from one end of the airplane to the other to stimulate my blood circulation. As I pace, I occasionally play a guessing game and ask myself which of the passengers seated on either side of the aisle suffers from sleep disordered breathing.

Extremely obese people with a short, thick neck, or a small and sunken lower jaw, and people who have fallen asleep with their mouths wide open are awarded particularly high marks in my guessing game, especially if they are middle-aged men. I am convinced that any sleep doctor can quickly picture the typical patient, who is easily recognizable anywhere, anytime. The main risk factors for the syndrome are obesity, narrowing of the upper airways, hereditary conditions, being an adult male, old age, and several specific diseases. Each of these factors contributes an independent risk to the syndrome.

Their Paunches Go Before Them

Dickens undoubtedly made his mark on the world of medicine, but he was not the first to observe the connection between obesity and sleepiness. William Shakespeare preceded him by almost 250 years. Sir John

Falstaff, young Prince Henry's partner in youthful mischief and one of Shakespeare's most popular characters, was known for his corpulence. According to Prince Henry, Falstaff was "this bed-presser, this horse back-breaker, this huge hill of flesh . . . that swollen parcel of dropsies, that huge bombard of sack, that stuffed cloak-bag of guts, that roasted Manningtree ox with the pudding in his belly" (*King Henry IV,* Part I). Falstaff, though, was also known for his propensity for napping in strange and unusual places. We see him sprawled, dozing in the middle of the day on a bench in the waiting room at Westminster Palace, and later in the play at the Boar's Head Tavern he is "fast asleep behind the arras, and snorting like a horse." Falstaff's breathing during sleep is indeed strange, as Prince Henry observes: "Hark, how hard he fetches breath." It may be, then, that it would be more historically accurate to call the syndrome characterizing obese and sleepy people the "Falstaff syndrome," or the "Henry IV syndrome," and not necessarily the Pickwickian syndrome.

Although thin people are also liable to suffer from sleep disordered breathing, it is much more common in obese people. What is the definition of obesity? We usually think of a person's weight in terms of kilograms or pounds, but this weight alone may be misleading. Eighty kilograms in a person 1.6 meters tall is not the same as that weight in a person 1.9 meters tall. The accepted unit in scientific literature to express weight in relation to height is body mass index (BMI), which is defined as body weight divided by height squared (kilograms per meter squared, or Kg/m^2). The body mass of the first person, the shorter of the two, is $31.25\ Kg/m^2$ by this calculation, whereas the body mass of the taller one is $22.1\ Kg/m^2$. According to criteria of the World Health Organization (WHO), body mass is divided into six classifications: BMI of less than 18.5 is defined as underweight; between 18.5 and 24.9 as normal weight; 25 to 29.9 as overweight; 30 to 34.9 as Grade 1 obesity; 35 to 39.9 as Grade 2 obesity; and over 40 as Grade 3 obesity.

Applying this measure of body mass to people with sleep apnea is revealing. Of the more than thirty thousand patients who have been diagnosed so far at the Technion Sleep Laboratory with sleep apnea syndrome, 82 percent were rated overweight or worse on the BMI scale, and

37 percent suffered from Grade 1, 2, or 3 obesity. The body mass of only 18 percent of those examined was normal. Although we do not know with certainty the syndrome's prevalence in all people with Grade 1, 2, or 3 obesity, based on our experience and that of others, it is possible that it could be as many as one in every three or four people!

The connection between body mass and sleep apnea syndrome is evident not only in a higher incidence of the syndrome in obese people but also in its severity, as measured by the average number of full or partial apneas per hour. In people whose body mass is normal the number of episodes per hour of sleep is only sixteen, whereas in those with Grade 1 obesity it is almost double that, at thirty episodes per hour. In people with Grade 3 obesity the figure is tripled, at forty-five episodes per hour.

The connection between obesity and the number of apneas during sleep is not limited to those who either requested or were referred by their doctor for examination at a sleep laboratory. It exists in people randomly sampled from the general population. This connection was investigated in the sample of Wisconsin civil servants, who were given a second sleep examination four years after their first. In those who had gained weight between the first and second examinations, the number of apneas had also increased, whereas in those who had lost weight, the number of apneas had decreased. The findings were unequivocal: a variation of 10 percent in body weight led to a change of some 30 percent in the number of apneas during sleep. Furthermore, among those whose body weight had increased by more than 10 percent, the probability of finding average to severe sleep breathing disorders increased sixfold.

Although we do not ordinarily distinguish between different types of obesity, accumulation of fatty tissue in the body tends to be inconsistent. Some people are fat only in the upper part of their body, in others it is their paunches that precede them, whereas in another group it is the legs and buttocks that are heavy. The greatest risk for breathing disorders during sleep is associated with weight gain in the upper part of the body, especially around the neck, chest, and stomach. The reason is that such weight gain causes narrowing of the upper airways and significantly impedes the functioning of the respiratory muscles and diaphragm. Sophisticated imaging techniques have shown that even sleep apnea syn-

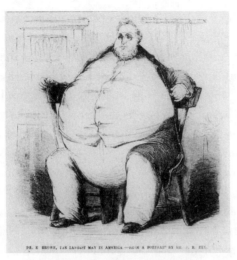

Dr. H. Brown, the fattest man in the
United States; a nineteenth-century
picture by J. R. Dix

drome patients who are not particularly obese are more prone to accumulation of fatty tissue around the neck than other people of the same body mass who do not have the syndrome. The upper airways in obese people or people with thick necks are unstable both during wakefulness and sleep. The connection between obesity and sleep apnea has far-reaching significance for the number of people who will experience severe sleep apnea syndrome in the future, especially in the United States, where several studies indicate that the prevalence of obesity is reaching epidemic proportions. During the 1990s, the percentage of adults with a body mass index higher than 30 almost doubled, from 12 percent in 1991 to 18.9 percent in 1999.

The increase is in both men and women, of all ethnic groups, irrespective of education or income levels. According to a study published in 1999 in the *Journal of the American Medical Association,* or *JAMA,* 15 percent of the population in only four of the forty-five states that participated in the 1991 survey had a body mass index of more than 30. In 1999 this number had increased to thirty-nine states. In sixteen states,

20 percent were obese! In a number of states the increase was alarming: in Georgia, an increase of 100 percent was recorded, in New Mexico 89 percent, and in Virginia 80 percent. Tourists visiting the United States cannot help noticing the large number of "heavyweights" who tip the scales at about 150 kilograms or even more. They can be seen on the street, in stores, at amusement parks, and especially in the "all you can eat" restaurants. It is cause for concern that American society is adapting to the change in its proportions: obesity is gaining legitimacy in special television programs for overweight people, in special magazines such as *FAT!SO?* as well as in publicity campaigns for equal civil rights for "heavy" people.

If the number of obese people continues to grow at the same rate, in fifty years at least half the population of the United States will have a body mass index higher than 30. The effect of increasing numbers of obese people on the prevalence of sleep apnea syndrome can be easily forecast. Since one in every three or four obese people also suffers from sleep disordered breathing, and as the severity of the syndrome increases with body weight, the number of sleep apnea patients in the United States is liable to reach huge proportions over the coming years.

Bird Face

As described earlier, the upper airways play an essential role in breathing control during sleep. Hence, it is hardly surprising that the second most important risk factor for sleep disordered breathing is narrowing of the upper airways. There are several causes of this kind of narrowing, including excess fatty tissue (which is the case with obese people), tumors around the pharynx, enlarged tonsils, and congenital facial structure characterized by a small and sunken chin. All of these can cause breathing disorders during sleep in certain people.

Narrowing of the upper airways is a risk factor for apneas during sleep for a simple reason: a physics principle called the Bernoulli effect. The upper airways can be likened to a long, narrow pipe connecting the lungs to the outer world through the nose and mouth. If the aperture of this pipe is constricted, the negative pressure created in the thorax when

inhaling will lead to collapse of the pipe's walls and blockage at its nar-
rowest point. This is easily demonstrated. If we inhale through a plastic
drinking straw, it will serve us well as long as it is not creased. If we make
a crease in it, for example by folding and unfolding it, its walls will adhere to each other as soon as we inhale and the straw will be blocked.
The crease will form at the fold. The upper airways are not straight and
smooth like a drinking straw, but more like a narrow, winding canyon in
which water has carved steep and rocky cliffs. The nose, the primary airway during sleep, is the most narrow and winding segment. Even in large
and prominent noses, the airway is no wider than a narrow crack of three
to five millimeters—which explains why so many people have chronically "blocked noses." The flow of air through the nose can be disrupted
because of fluid secretions or ones that have solidified because of abnor-
mality of the nasal septum or enlargement of the nasal turbinate. Even
when airflow has a smooth passage through the nose, it may come up
against a huge tongue or enlarged tonsils, thickened pharyngeal walls,
collapsed loose tissue in the soft palate (the rear section of the palate), or
a large uvula (the conical fleshy body suspended from the middle of the
soft palate, the main function of which is to prevent the flow of fluids
from the oral cavity into the nasal passages).

As long as we are awake, the tonus of the smooth muscles in the
upper airways is high, so the airways are kept open. As noted earlier, during wakefulness muscle tonus in sleep apnea patients is higher than in
healthy people, to compensate for narrower airways. However, this situation changes during sleep. First, since we sleep lying down, and many
do so on their backs, the soft tissue tends to collapse and block the airways even more. Second, during sleep the tonus of the smooth muscles
slackens, increasing even more the tendency of the soft tissue to collapse
and block the airways. It is highly probable that the slackening of the
smooth muscles during sleep is even greater in sleep apnea patients, although the reason for this is not yet known.

Consequently, it is little wonder that an ear, nose, and throat examination of sleep apnea patients produces an abundance of findings. An
abnormal nasal septum, enlarged tonsils, a large and thickened uvula, or
a huge tongue blocking the oral cavity and leaving only a narrow passage

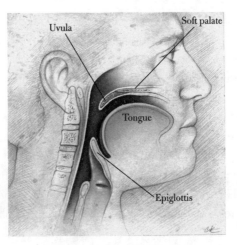

The back of the throat, showing
particularly the location of the uvula,
a major contributor to snoring and apneas.
The airways become obstructed more
easily when lying down, as at right,
especially if the soft palate or tongue is
large or the person has a receding jaw.
(Illustration © Christy Krames)

for air can be found in many of them. Use of modern imaging techniques
to describe the facial skeleton reveals characteristics unique to sleep apnea
patients. Some present a narrow and sunken chin, which gives their face
in profile a form suggesting a "bird's face"; others have a low palate or a
small, sunken lower jaw.

Although collapse of the airways does not occur in the nose, modern research has corroborated Catlin's ideas regarding the essential role
of nasal breathing during sleep. Nasal breathing has two unique characteristics that distinguish it from mouth breathing. First, the nose functions as a heating element. The air passing through the nose is slightly
warmed and reaches the lungs at a temperature more comfortable for the
body. Second, the nose functions as a filter for dust particles and other
pollutants that are inhaled from the air, as Galen pointed out two thou-

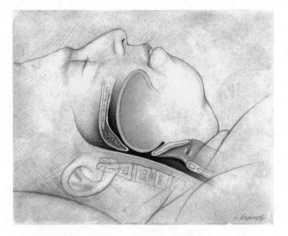

sand years ago. Furthermore, as we have seen, there are special sensors in the nose that relay information to the brain's respiratory center on airflow passing over them. Using these sensors, the nose actively participates in controlling and managing respiration. Local anesthesia that neutralizes these sensors causes disruption of the respiratory center's activity during sleep.

Another simple method proving that nose breathing during sleep is essential is to block the nostrils. Whether the nose is blocked mechanically or as a result of a chronic cold, the result is the same: disruption of the respiratory center's activity and suspensions of breathing. Tests at the sleep laboratory have shown this both in people who have allergic colds and in completely healthy people who have their noses blocked during sleep by sealing their nostrils with adhesive tape. In both cases, the patients experienced full or partial apneas that always culminated in a brief awakening. We do not have an unequivocal answer why the activity of the brain's respiratory center is disrupted when airflow in the nose is blocked, but there are at least two possibilities: One, blocking the nose possibly puts the airflow sensors out of action, similar to the effect of local anesthesia on the nostrils. Two, since people are accustomed to breathe through their nose during sleep, they try to breathe through it despite the blockage, hence significantly increasing the nega-

tive pressure in the thorax. Consequently, if there is a narrowing somewhere in the upper airways, the pressure will lead, according to the
Bernoulli principle, to a collapse at the point of narrowing, resulting in
apneas during sleep.

In view of modern findings on the importance of breathing
through the nose during sleep, it is hard not to be amazed at George
Catlin's keen perception when he claimed more than a century ago that
it is the key to healthy sleep and longevity.

Generations of Snorers

The experience of many sleep researchers shows that snoring fathers
have snoring children, as can be seen from the following case. About
twenty years ago, when every new sleep apnea patient diagnosed at the
laboratory still aroused great excitement, the sleep technician called me
in the middle of the night to come and see "something remarkable." Indeed, I was greatly surprised when instead of leading me to the recording instruments, the technician led me to the waiting room, where the
son of the patient being examined that night was fast asleep in an armchair. The son was choking and suffocating in his sleep just like his
father who was sleeping in the nearby bedroom, hooked up to the recording instruments. We awakened the son and after a brief interview
discovered that this was an unusual family. There were six girls and six
boys, and all the boys snored and choked in their sleep, but not one of
the girls did. Since the patient's son was a taxi driver by profession, we
arranged for him to bring all his brothers and sisters in his taxi to be examined at the laboratory. The examinations revealed sleep apnea of varying severity in each of his brothers but in none of his sisters.

Although this family was unusual, it was not the only one of its
kind. Over the years we have come across many relatives, mostly fathers
and sons, who have sleep apnea syndrome, usually at similar levels of
severity. In exhaustive interviews we conducted with large numbers of
sleep apnea patients, a quarter of them reported an additional family
member with the syndrome. In 70 percent of cases, it was a parent, and in

30 percent a brother or sister. Similar evidence of a familial tendency toward snoring and sleep apnea has also been recorded in other parts of the world. Several studies have even shown that snoring is hereditary. Salvatore Smirne's group from Milan compared the snoring habits of 492 identical twins with those of 284 fraternal twins. The researchers found that when one sibling was a chronic snorer, there was a higher probability that his identical twin would snore too than was the case with fraternal twins. The main factors leading to snoring in fraternal twins were body weight, respiratory diseases, and smoking. A Danish study that examined snoring habits in 3,387 men in Copenhagen found that one of the important indicators of the existence of chronic snoring was a family history of chronic snorers. According to the study's findings, all the men in Copenhagen who had been forced out of the master bedroom by their female bedfellows because of snoring had a family history of snoring. In 23 percent of them, it was the father, and in 10 percent the mother. In contrast, only 8 percent of the non-snorers described their fathers as chronic snorers, and only 3.4 percent described their mothers this way.

A milestone in our approach to the hereditary factor in sleep apnea syndrome was a study we conducted with children of syndrome patients. After we discovered that obstruction of the nose during sleep causes frequent apneas and awakenings, we decided to examine the sons of syndrome patients. Our assumption was that if there is a genetic factor for sleep disordered breathing, obstructing the nose of sleep apnea patients' children would cause even more severe breathing disorders during sleep than in a control group. For the purpose of the study, we blocked the airflow through the nose during sleep in six children of sleep apnea syndrome patients. Without exception, all the children whose noses had been blocked experienced a large number of apneas during sleep. The average number of apneas increased tenfold with the obstruction, from one per hour to ten, whereas in the control group the increase was more moderate, from one apnea to three. It seemed that when the noses of the patients' children were blocked, their brain's respiratory center stopped functioning normally and started faltering. Their reaction to the experiment itself was dramatic. They reported that they had difficulty breathing through their mouths, and two of them woke up in the middle with an alarming feeling of suffocation and asked to stop the experiment. Not one of them was prepared to repeat the experiment.

Dr. Giora Pillar, one of the talented sleep researchers to come out of the Technion's sleep laboratory, provided a possible answer for why obstruction of the nose led to such severe breathing disorders in patients' children. Many of my colleagues in the world of sleep research wonder how we have achieved such rapid and successful developments in sleep medicine in a country as small as Israel. One of the reasons is our success in recruiting a team of talented and dedicated doctors and technicians who spend day and night in the laboratory researching and conducting examinations. The team of technicians usually includes medical students recruited for night work immediately after being accepted to medical school. Medical studies in Israel last six years, and the students spend one or two nights a week during this period at the Technion's sleep laboratories in Haifa, Tel Aviv, Holon, Hadera, and Jerusalem. Those who develop an interest in sleep research and sleep medicine during this period join the laboratory team when they graduate, becoming full partners in the clinical and research work. Upon completion of their studies, the others, due to their prolonged exposure to the field, serve as faithful ambassadors for sleep medicine wherever they go.

Dr. Giora Pillar followed this course. He started out during his first year of studies as a technician. When he graduated from medical school and completed his specialization in pediatrics, he joined the laboratory team at the Technion. Prior to that, he spent two years of advanced study at Harvard University's sleep laboratory. For his doctoral dissertation, Giora researched the family factor in sleep apnea syndrome. He persuaded ninety men and women, from forty-five families in which either the father or the mother had been diagnosed with the syndrome, to be examined at the sleep laboratory. Their ages ranged from sixteen to fifty-two. The sleep records showed that 47 percent of patients' children were afflicted with sleep disordered breathing, whereas a further 22 percent were chronic snorers. In 13 percent of the people tested, the examinations showed more than thirty apneas per hour, indicating a moderate to severe level of the syndrome. In three-quarters of the patients' children, who were over the age of thirty-five, the prevalence of sleep apnea was twelve times greater than in the general population.

We were unaware that at the very same time a group from Cleveland was conducting a similar study that showed identical findings, and it happened that the studies from Cleveland and Haifa, both reporting that sleep apnea syndrome is significantly more prevalent in children of people with the syndrome than in the general population, were published in the same issue of the *American Review of Respiratory Diseases*. These findings reinforced the hypothesis that, in at least some cases, the background for sleep breathing disorders is genetic.

But what is it that patients' children inherit that has such a significant effect on their breathing during sleep? Could it be a unique facial structure, like a small jaw or a large uvula, that causes narrowing of the upper airways? Perhaps it is a physique with a tendency to weight gain around the neck? Or perhaps the genetic factor is the disruption of the respiratory center's function itself? It is known that each of these elements is influenced by hereditary factors. However, examinations of the upper airways in patients' children did not show any unusual findings. There was no irregularity in their facial structure, and we detected no particular tendency toward obesity in them. Nevertheless, our previous findings on the effect of blocking the nose during sleep in patients' children gave rise to another possibility: that the genetic factor is connected to the respiratory center's ability to deal with changes in the airways' resistance during sleep.

The term "resistance" denotes the total resistance to airflow in the upper airways. Clearly, the narrower the airways, the greater the resistance to airflow. Most of us, in response to changes in resistance, are capable of performing the required adjustments to maintain regular breathing during sleep by accelerating breathing rhythm or depth, or by heightening the tonus of the smooth muscles in the airways. For some, however, every change in resistance causes imbalance and irregular functioning of the brain's respiratory center, and consequently the airways are completely blocked.

To test this hypothesis Pillar conducted a further experiment. After completing the first study on the syndrome's prevalence in patients' children, he recruited ten of the patients' children who were of sound health during the sleep examination, and asked them to sleep in the laboratory again. This time, however, they were required to breathe through a mask placed over their noses and connected to an air pipe with an adjustable valve. Using the valve, the pipe's opening could be gradually narrowed, increasing resistance to airflow in a controlled manner. When the recording instruments indicated that the patient had fallen asleep, Giora slowly increased the resistance to airflow, necessitating gradual intensification of respiratory exertion from the patients. The results of the increased resistance were dissimilar in children of sleep apnea patients and a control group composed of boys and girls of the same age group without a family history of breathing disorders during sleep. Those in the control group increased the rhythm of their breathing and deepened it in response to increased resistance. But in the patients' children, who you will recall were completely healthy and did not even snore, the increase in resistance led to the appearance of partial apneas during sleep. In other words, the patients' children were unable to perform the adjustments required to efficiently deal with the increased resistance to airflow unless they first awoke from their sleep. The results of the study led to the conclusion that at least one of the genetic factors for sleep apnea syndrome is connected to the ability of the brain's respiratory center to sense changes in resistance to airflow during sleep and perform the required adjustments in smooth muscle tonus, and in the rhythm and depth of breathing. The respiratory center in some people is not sensitive to these changes, so they are unable to perform adjustments to their breathing, and consequently their breathing during sleep is disrupted.

It later transpired that disruption in the regulation of breathing among relatives of sleep apnea patients does not occur only during sleep. The research group in Cleveland, led by Susan Redline, proved that relatives of sleep apnea patients do not respond normally to respiratory stimuli during wakefulness either. The response of patients' relatives to a drop in oxygen concentration in air inhaled during wakefulness was less vigorous than that of the control group. We do not yet know whether in relatives of sleep apnea patients the disruption in the respiratory center's activity is due to failure of the sensors to relay information on airflow in the upper airways, or failure of the chemical sensors to relay information on quantities of oxygen and carbon dioxide, or the respiratory center's failure to process the information relayed to it. Another possibility is that disruption occurs in the function of the corrective mechanism, which is controlled by the muscles that expand the airways and by increasing the activity of the respiratory muscles. Further research is required to investigate these possibilities.

Additional confirmation that genetic factors play a role in increasing the risk of contracting the symptom can be found in studies of the variance in the syndrome's prevalence and severity in different ethnic groups. Initial findings reported on the African-American population, with the Redline group from Cleveland again making a significant contribution. It found that African-Americans have a greater risk of contracting sleep apnea syndrome than do Caucasians. This risk was particularly high among youths up to age eighteen—three-and-a-half times that of Caucasians the same age. These findings could not be explained by variances in body weight or other factors such as smoking or alcohol intake. Furthermore, in African-American children who suffered from sleep disordered breathing, the syndrome was more severe than in Caucasian or Hispanic children. Similar findings were revealed in African-American adults over sixty-five, compared with Caucasians of the same age.

A similar comparative study was conducted in Singapore, a country whose diverse population includes a large number of ethnic groups. Sleep apnea syndrome is more prevalent in Singaporeans of Malay origin than in those of Chinese or Indian origin. In this study, too, it was impossible to associate the variance in the syndrome's prevalence with differences in body weight or neck circumference. It is interesting that in a comparison conducted at Stanford University's sleep laboratory between sleep apnea patients of Chinese and European origin, it was the patients of Chinese origin who had more severe sleep apnea syndrome. Double the number of Chinese-origin patients, compared with those of European origin, were classified as "severe" and had more than fifty apneas in one hour of sleep. Since the Chinese are not renowned for heavy body weight or thick necks, clearly the reasons need to be sought in other genetic factors. Some suggested that this may be related to the fact that the geometry of the base of the skull is different in Asians from the Far East than in Caucasians, which results in narrower airways and therefore in more severe sleep apnea.

Another example comes from the Pacific. Anyone happening upon the exotic Pacific Islands cannot help noticing the dimensions of the islanders. The Maoris, the original inhabitants of New Zealand, the Tongans, the Aborigines, and other island inhabitants of the Pacific Ocean have a particularly heavy physique featuring a thick neck and a broad chest. The sleep laboratory in Oakland, New Zealand, reported that the prevalence of sleep apnea syndrome in patients of Maori origin and native islanders of the Pacific Ocean is double that of patients of European origin. In this instance, the high prevalence of the syndrome is probably connected to the physique of the native islanders.

Men Snore and Women Toss and Turn

When I returned to Israel from the United States in 1975, I established a two-bed sleep laboratory at the Technion in Haifa, the initial function of which was research. As soon as word got out that I was engaged in "sleep examinations," however, relatives, neighbors, and friends started pleading with me to examine or advise them or their acquaintances with sleep disorders of every kind. So it came to pass that the inaugural sleep apnea syndrome diagnosis at the Technion's sleep laboratory was that of H.W., a stocky, plump woman with a rare sense of humor, who joked about her amazing capacity to fall asleep anywhere, anytime. An acquaintance of hers asked me to examine her "just to find out why she sleeps all the time." My curiosity was piqued after he told me that H.W. had fallen asleep as she was ironing her laundry and the hot iron had started a fire in her home. At our first meeting, H.W. told me that her doctors had explained that high levels of carbon dioxide in her blood caused her to fall asleep—the customary explanation for sleepiness in Pickwickian patients at the time.

The nocturnal examination showed that H.W. was a person with severe sleep apnea syndrome. She had hundreds of apneas that began as soon as she fell asleep. My feelings following H.W.'s examination were similar to the excitement and satisfaction I felt in San Diego after seeing my first sleep apnea patient. I realized anew that the sleep examination had discovered something that could not have been found any other way. Since H.W.'s doctor, Gideon Elroy, was one of my colleagues at the Technion Faculty of Medicine, I reported my findings to him. To my great surprise, not only did Dr. Elroy not cast any doubt on the results of the exam, he reacted with real enthusiasm. He asked me to come over to his office at the hospital, immediately if possible, and to bring the sleep records so that he could see the apneas with his own eyes. The reason for his enthusiasm soon became apparent. In 1956, Elroy and a colleague had reported on a poulterer who would fall asleep at the counter in his store, and who made a complete recovery following a tracheostomy. Like all Pickwickian patients at the time, the poulterer's sleepiness was explained as carbon dioxide poisoning. Now the real reasons for his complaint had been uncovered. This meeting led to a long friendship with a doctor who believed in the clinical importance of the syndrome at a time when most of his colleagues completely ignored it.

I do not know how many sleep laboratories were inaugurated by an examination of a woman with sleep apnea, but it may be safely assumed that the number is very small. The reason for this is that sleep apnea syndrome is much more prevalent in men, a fact expressed even in folklore. Caricatures of loud snoring, one of the most obvious signs of suspensions of breathing during sleep, usually describe the suffering of women, who toss and turn in their beds, unable to fall asleep because of their partner's loud trumpeting snores. There are no such caricatures describing similar experiences among men. One of the most common scenes in a laboratory for diagnosis of sleep disorders is of a husband and wife coming for consultation, the woman clutching her husband's elbow and dragging him, almost against his will, to the sleep doctor's office. In the meeting with the doctor she describes her predicament and announces that she can no longer stand the nightly torture of her husband's snoring. He, on the other hand, usually emphatically denies the possibility that he snores and chokes in his sleep and claims that it is all a figment of his wife's highly developed imagination.

The accumulated experience of sleep laboratories throughout the world shows that eight to ten times more men than women suffer from sleep apnea. Moreover, when the syndrome is compared in men and women of the same age and body mass, it transpires that it is also more severe in men. Our observations with thousands of sleep apnea patients illustrate this clearly. Women experience fewer sleep apneas than men do, irrespective of body mass or age. The most striking difference is in the thirty-to-forty age group, where the men averaged twenty-seven apneas per hour, and the women had an average of eighteen. The male patients with Grade 1 obesity experienced more than thirty episodes per hour, the females more than twenty; similarly, in Grade 2 obesity the males have forty apneas per hour and females twenty-five. Furthermore, the saturation values of arterial oxygen during sleep are lower in men than in women, which is also an indication of the syndrome's severity. The distribution by age of men and women with the syndrome varies, with the largest number, relatively speaking, of males between forty and fifty, and the largest number of women between fifty and sixty.

Can the variance in age distribution between men and women teach us something about the reasons for the difference in the syndrome's prevalence and severity? The increase in the number of women over fifty who live with the syndrome indicates that the difference between the sexes may be hormonal. During their reproductive period, which usually ends around age fifty, women secrete high levels of the female sex hormones progesterone and estrogen. Since it is known that progesterone has a stimulating influence on breathing functions, it may be that until the end of menstruation progesterone secretion protects against breathing disorders during sleep. This protection is reduced when the levels of progesterone decrease drastically after menstruation ceases. As we will see later, based on this hypothesis experimenters have tried progesterone treatments on men with sleep disordered breathing, but these have proved unsuccessful.

The male sex hormone, testosterone, also plays a role in variations between the sexes. Sleep examinations in men with testosterone deficiency showed apneas during sleep only after they were treated with the hormone. There have also been reports of women with high levels of testosterone, usually due to ovarian tumors, who had breathing disorders during sleep. These completely disappeared after testosterone levels were reduced to normal. Hence it is possible that both progesterone and testosterone affect respiratory function during sleep, and any change in their levels or the balance between them may cause disruption to respiratory functions during sleep.

The difference between the sexes in respiratory function during sleep is not limited to sleep apnea syndrome. Studies have shown that women are more resistant than men to upper airway collapse during sleep. When Giora Pillar completed his doctoral studies in my laboratory, he went on to advanced postdoctoral studies in David White's laboratory at Harvard, taking with him the device he had used to examine the effect of airflow resistance changes in the nostrils on the breathing functions of sleep apnea patients' children. In White's laboratory, he used the instrument to investigate whether there is a difference between the sexes in responses to airflow resistance changes during sleep. Although an increase in resistance to airflow caused partial apneas in both men and women, they appeared at significantly higher resistance values in women than in men, making it appear that the adjustment mechanisms to increases in resistance to airflow are more efficient in women than in men. Recently, White's group demonstrated that men have a larger soft palate, which is the area most vulnerable to collapse in the upper airways. This also points to a mechanical difference between men and women. There is, therefore, a solid physiological basis for women experiencing sleep apnea syndrome less than men do.

A number of years earlier, White showed that during wakefulness, too, women enjoy airways that are more stable and resistant to collapse than do men. He measured the activity of the smooth muscles in the upper airways during inhalation and found that muscle activity in women was more intensive than in men.

In spite of the consensus that sleep apnea is significantly more prevalent in men than in women, some claim that the impression obtained in sleep laboratories accentuates the differences. In epidemiological studies investigating the syndrome's prevalence in the general population, such as the study of Wisconsin civil servants, the ratio between the sexes is closer to 1:3 or 1:4, rather than 1:8 or 1:10, which is the data from populations examined in sleep laboratories. There are several possible reasons for the variance between laboratory examinations and population studies. First, women with sleep apnea syndrome may suffer from snoring and daytime sleepiness, the two most prominent signs of the syndrome, less than men do. Second, women may be more embarrassed to admit that they snore, hence they do not complain to their doctors. Third, sleep examinations are possibly less accessible to women than they are to men, and there are examples of such a difference in other fields of medicine, too.

Another possibility is that the nature of the complaints by women with sleep disordered breathing differs from that of men. To test this, we randomly selected a group of 650 women and 650 men from the sleep apnea patients who had been diagnosed at the Technion Sleep Laboratory. We compared their complaints of snoring, daytime sleepiness and frequent awakenings, daytime fatigue, morning headaches, difficulties in falling asleep, and morning fatigue. We also examined how these complaints were connected to the level of severity of sleep breathing disorders. Analysis of the complaints showed significant differences between the sexes, especially in the young and the old. Whereas women up to age forty with sleep apnea complained only about snoring, men of the same age complained equally about snoring, daytime sleepiness, and frequent awakenings. Between ages forty and sixty, men and women alike complained about snoring and restless sleep, but the men also complained about daytime sleepiness. Snoring, therefore, is a common complaint of both men and women with sleep disordered breathing, but the complaint about daytime sleepiness is more characteristic of men. Since the combination of excessive sleepiness and loud snoring is a symptom of the syndrome, it is easy to understand why fewer women are referred for diagnosis at sleep laboratories. Therefore, it is necessary to pay more attention to women's complaints about loud snoring in order to diagnose the syndrome in them.

From the Sleep of a Baby to the Sleep of the Elderly

The connection between age and sleep apnea has been the subject of lively debate among numerous researchers for the past several years. It is known and agreed that the risk of sleep apnea is not identical in the different age groups. Breathing disorders during sleep are more prevalent in children than in youths, and with the exception of individual cases they are rarely diagnosed before the age of twenty-five to thirty. The syndrome's prevalence gradually increases between the twenties and sixties, and then decreases again. There are few cases of women prior to menopause, at which point the number of cases rises significantly. We are unable to explain why the syndrome's prevalence from the teen years up to the end of the second decade of life is so low. Some claim that the gradual increase is evidence that age is a risk factor for sleep disordered breathing that is not contingent on other factors. Their explanation is that as a person gets older, breathing during sleep is less and less stable.

Some years ago, we studied the connection between secretion of melatonin—a hormone secreted by the pineal gland, which is located in the depths of the brain and is known to affect sleep regulation—and the quality of sleep in the elderly. For this we required a sample of twenty healthy people who were seventy or older. To recruit volunteers, we spent quite some time in retirement homes and golden-age clubs in the Haifa area. Those who were eligible and agreed to participate in the study were asked to spend a night at the sleep laboratory to assess the qualities of their sleep. We were in for a surprise. Although all the volunteers had reported in interviews that their sleep was normal, the sleep recordings showed breathing disorders during sleep in almost all of them. In fact, in half of them the recordings found more than ten apneas per hour—which is the accepted threshold for the syndrome's diagnosis in adults. I particularly remember an amiable man of about eighty who was energetic and alert during the day, although our examination had recorded some 200 apneas during his sleep. He dismissed the possibility that he suffered from any sleep disorder whatsoever.

Apneas during sleep that are not accompanied by complaints of fatigue or sleepiness are characteristic not only of the elderly in Haifa—they have been reported in other places too, although their significance is still controversial. In the study of Wisconsin civil servants, 25 percent of men experienced at least five full or partial apneas per hour, whereas only 10 percent also complained of daytime sleepiness. Furthermore, similar to our experiment in melatonin research, there is ample evidence that laboratory findings of sleep disordered breathing in the elderly are not accompanied by daytime fatigue, sleepiness, or diminishing mental abilities. In addition, sleep apnea is linked with risk of hypertension and cardiovascular disease in young people, but not among the elderly. Perhaps some suspensions of breathing during sleep are normal in the elderly and do not indicate sleep apnea syndrome, a conclusion that would require different classifications for the syndrome in different age groups.

Disease as a Risk Factor for Sleep Apnea

Several diseases increase the risk for sleep apnea syndrome; some are connected to changes in metabolic activity, others to blockage of the airways or the respiratory muscles. Among the major diseases connected to the syndrome are kidney disease, acromegaly, heart disease, and thyroid deficiency.

Kidney Disease

Sleep disorders are very common in kidney disease patients. Most of them complain of disturbed night sleep or considerable daytime sleepiness. In sleep records of kidney disease patients on dialysis treatment, it was found that they experience two main disorders: periodic leg movements in sleep (restless legs syndrome) and sleep apnea syndrome. Half the patients suffered from sleep apnea syndrome. The reasons for this are insufficiently clear. One possibility is that the change in blood gas levels and especially a drop in the carbon dioxide level may cause periodic breathing, leading to central apneas or even obstructive apneas. A second possibility is that the accumulation of fluids in the upper airways due to kidney malfunction may narrow the air passage and cause it to collapse during sleep. Furthermore, laxity of the smooth muscles in the upper airways as a result of neural damage may also aggravate the susceptibility to collapse. Although the mechanism causing the apneas is not known in detail, the fact that successful kidney transplant patients have dramatically improved breathing functions during sleep proves a direct connection between kidney diseases and breathing disorders. Patrick Hanly and Andreas Pierratos of Toronto recently reported that dialysis patients receiving treatment during the night experienced a significant improvement in respiratory functions during sleep: during nocturnal dialysis, the number of apneas dropped from an average of forty-six per hour to only nine. When dialysis was done during the day, no change in apneas during the patients' sleep was observed. The researchers presumed that the primary reason for the dramatic change in respiratory functions in sleep during dialysis was stabilization of blood gas levels.

Did Goliath Suffer from Sleep Apnea Syndrome?

Acromegaly is a chronic disease caused by excessive secretion of growth hormone, which causes enlargement of the organs and increases the risk of arthritic diseases, diabetes, hypertension, and heart disease. The mortality rate of acromegaly patients is twice to three times greater than that of the general population. It has been known for many years that patients with acromegaly are also prone to daytime sleepiness; some people maintain that acromegaly patients often suffer from narcolepsy. But sleep laboratory examinations show that they are actually enduring sleep apnea. According to a survey conducted recently among fifty-five acromegaly patients in Czechoslovakia, about 75 percent of them had sleep apnea syndrome. Researchers reported that the patients' neck circumference was the factor indicating presence of the syndrome. In Germany, sleep apnea syndrome was detected in 40 percent of acromegaly patients, and in this study, too, neck circumference was the primary indicator. In a comparison between acromegaly patients who suffer from sleep apnea and others that do not, variances were also recorded in facial structure, with differences in the structure of the lower jaw leaving a narrower passage for air.

Whether sleep apnea in acromegaly patients is connected to the disease itself or to its results is not certain. A number of studies indicate that in some cases sleep breathing disorders are directly connected to excessive secretion of growth hormone. For example, in cases where the cause of growth hormone secretion was a tumor on the pituitary gland, surgical removal of the tumor resulted in improvement of respiratory functions during sleep without intervention in facial structure or the airways. Treatment by medication to prevent secretion of growth hormone also resulted in a significant improvement in respiratory functions during sleep, although this improvement was not consistent in all the patients. In some, the hormone level was reduced, but there was no improvement in their breathing, whereas in others only a partial reduction of the hormone level led to total disappearance of sleep disordered breathing.

Some have conjectured that Goliath the Philistine, who David vanquished with a stone from a sling, suffered from acromegaly. If this is true, then it is possible that he also suffered from sleep apnea, and it may be assumed that his daytime sleepiness was an impediment in his battle against the alert and agile David.

Heart Failure

"Heart disease" is the popular term for a condition in which the heart is unable to provide the body's oxygen requirements. There can be several reasons for the heart's failure, such as a disease that damages its valves or the arteries feeding blood to the cardiac muscle itself (atherosclerosis of the coronary arteries), hypertension, alcoholism, diabetes, or viral damage. Of them all, atherosclerosis of the coronary arteries and hypertension are the most common. When the oxygen supply to the cardiac muscle is disrupted due to an obstruction in the coronary arteries, the force of its contraction is reduced and the amount of blood flowing from it is insufficient to feed oxygen to the organs. In hypertension, the body's arteries contract and the heart has to function more vigorously for the blood to flow to all parts of the body. Although in many cases the heart is capable of performing the required adjustments, sometimes the increased burden leads to its malfunction. Consequently, the heart enlarges and has difficulty contracting normally. The symptoms a person with heart disease usually complains of are shortness of breath, excessive tiredness, and swelling of the feet and ankles, which is a result of fluid accumulation due to the heart's inability to ensure normal blood flow.

Hunter, Cheyne, and Stokes were the first to observe abnormal breathing in heart patients during sleep, and Stokes was the first to determine that breathing disorders during sleep are characteristic of heart patients. Sleep studies of heart patients have confirmed his conclusion. About half of these patients experience periodic breathing during sleep, now known as Cheyne-Stokes breathing. Using a metaphor from the world of music, Cheyne-Stokes breathing is described as crescendo-decrescendo patterns, referring to heightened intensity of breathing, which after climaxing decreases and gradually weakens until it stops completely for a few seconds before intensifying again.

Although Cheyne-Stokes breathing has been known for almost two hundred years, its clinical importance has only recently been recognized. Like sleep apnea patients, heart patients with Cheyne-Stokes breathing also awaken several times during sleep without being aware of it, especially during the crescendo, when breathing reaches the climax of its intensity. The oxygen and carbon dioxide levels in the blood rise and fall according to the changes in breathing intensity. Several studies have found that the life expectancy of heart patients who also suffer from Cheyne-Stokes breathing is lower than that of heart patients who do not. The variance between the two groups could not be explained, so it was assumed that either the breathing pattern itself or the awakenings and changes in blood gas levels accompanying it affect the heart patient's clinical condition. Effective treatment for breathing disorders during sleep has led to a significant improvement in the condition of heart patients and to longer life expectancy.

No exhaustive reasons have been found to explain why so many heart patients suffer from Cheyne-Stokes breathing during sleep. There is a tendency to associate the occurrence with the changes in the intensity and volume of blood flow in heart patients, especially in those whose respiratory center is particularly sensitive to concentration levels of carbon dioxide in the blood.

Hypoactivity of the Thyroid Gland

A deficiency in thyroxin, the hormone secreted by the thyroid gland, can be the result of gland malfunction or of a disease in the brain's pituitary gland or the hypothalamus, both of which regulate its activity. Patients with thyroid hypoactivity complain of excessive fatigue, sleepiness, and reduced intellectual abilities, all of which are also characteristic of sleep apnea patients. The similarity of the complaints and the fact that a thyroxin deficiency causes narrowing of the airways and possible malfunction of the brain's respiratory center gave rise to the hypothesis that hormonal disorders are a risk factor for sleep disordered breathing. Indeed, several studies, most of which were conducted on a small number of patients, found a relatively high prevalence of breathing disorders during sleep. Furthermore, in a number of cases, hormonal treatment led to improvement of sleep disordered breathing and the disappearance of complaints about fatigue and sleepiness. Most of the patients in whom severe sleep breathing disorders were observed, however, also experienced significant weight gain and did not respond to thyroxin treatment.

9

The Syndrome's Symptoms

The diagnosis of any illness begins with the patient's complaints, which provide the doctor with one end of a thread that will finally lead to an accurate diagnosis and appropriate treatment. As sleep apnea syndrome is manifested by suspensions of breathing during sleep, one might expect people afflicted with it to complain that they awaken from sleep because of shortness of breath or a suffocating sensation, but this is not so. People with the syndrome are totally oblivious of their nightly drama, they are usually very surprised to hear about it, and their response is something like, "But Doctor, I never wake up during the night." They sometimes reject the descriptions of suffocation provided by their partners so strongly that it causes family strife. Moreover, they never even dream about it.

Dr. Micha Gross collected more than two hundred dreams from sleep apnea patients after waking them from dream sleep in the laboratory. The subjects experienced apneas in all the sleep stages, including REM sleep. Gross found no evidence that sleep apnea syndrome patients dreamed about subjects linked to their breathing or breathing difficulties, any more than people who don't suffer from apneas. Accordingly, the patients' complaints reflect the results of the apneas and their accompanying awakenings, and not the episodes themselves.

To investigate what made sleep apnea patients seek help, we put the following question to 250 people with a particularly severe form of the syndrome: "Why did you come to the sleep laboratory for the first

Reasons given by sleep apnea patients for seeking help

I was told that my loud snoring was disturbing	79%
I woke up a number of times every night	55%
I was told that I stop breathing numerous times during sleep	54%
I felt constant physical tiredness	51%
I fell asleep numerous times during the day for no apparent reason	35%
I found it hard to concentrate at work	22%
I suffered from headaches in the mornings	21%
I was very irritable	21%
I fell asleep while driving on a few occasions	19%
I experienced difficulty in sexual intercourse	9%
I suffered from depression	9%

Note: Patients were allowed to give as many reasons as applied to them

time?" The reason that topped the list of their answers was loud snoring that disturbed the family: 79 percent of the patients said this was why they had come in for an evaluation. The next most common reasons were numerous awakenings from sleep (55 percent), stopping breathing during sleep, based on evidence from a family member (54 percent), and prolonged physical tiredness (51 percent). Thirty-five percent of the patients came to the laboratory because of their tendency to fall asleep during the day, and 19 percent because of falling asleep at the wheel. But sleep disorders are multifaceted, as the accompanying table shows, and there were also patients who noted morning headaches, great irritability, problems in sexual relations, or depression as the reasons that brought them to the laboratory for advice.

Everything About Snoring

Loud snoring is one of the most noticeable symptoms of sleep apnea syndrome. Although not every chronic snorer has sleep apnea syndrome, almost every person who has the syndrome is indeed a chronic snorer.

If the folkloristic preoccupation with snoring, the jokes and caricatures, are anything to go by, then snoring has troubled humankind since
the dawn of history. It can force a couple into separate bedrooms and
even into separate homes. In hospitals, snoring can cause a patient to be
banished from his bed in a ward to a remote room, while in the military
snorers are given a tent to themselves. Snoring often disturbs our sleep
just when we are in desperate need of it, after a hard day's work or an ex-
hausting hike.

I have heard innumerable stories about snoring, but the one that is
etched most clearly in my memory is an experience I had on a night flight
from Boston to London. As economy class was overbooked, I was up-
graded to a first-class seat and waited for takeoff with pleasurable expec-
tation. Much to my chagrin I soon realized that my upgrade was very
much a pig in a poke. Just before takeoff the captain welcomed aboard a
prominent member of the U.S. Senate who was a guest of honor aboard
the aircraft. The moment the aircraft took off, the guest of honor lay
down in his armchair—the jewel in the crown of that particular airline—
and his snores swiftly filled the small first-class compartment. His snoring was so loud that it drowned out the noise of the plane's engines. But
these were not normal snores—they were intermittent, and between
each series there was total silence that ended with sounds of choking and
suffocating. The sleeping senator, who was a very large man, immediately became the focus of attention of both passengers and cabin crew,
who all watched the phenomenon with astonishment. After a few minutes I was forced to pacify a frightened flight attendant who feared the
senator's imminent demise. I explained to her that this was how he had
been sleeping in his own bed for years and there was no reason for him
to leave this world during her tour of duty. And so we crossed the At-
lantic to the sounds of choking and suffocation that somehow resembled
the sound of a fuel-starved automobile engine. On landing in London I
buttonholed the purser and with a serious expression declared that the
company "owed" me a first-class flight. He agreed with me completely,
but explained politely that he was not authorized to make such a com-
mitment on the company's behalf.

It is no small wonder that we can find references to snoring and its
implications in the earliest periods of human history. Dio Chrysostom,

known as "Golden Mouth," who lived in Greece in the first century C.E., was, as his name implies, a gifted orator. Thirty-seven of his orations have survived and one, the thirty-third, is extraordinary in its content. It was delivered to the citizens of Tarsus in ancient Cilicia—today Antalya in Turkey, and identified by some as the biblical Tarshish—and it dealt almost exclusively with snoring. According to Chrysostom, the natives of Tarsus were wonderful people who spent all their time sleeping—whether sitting, standing, or walking, they were always sleeping. And how was their sleeping detected? By sleep's most typical sign: the sound of snoring. The people of Tarsus simply did not stop snoring, and this deplorable habit was common to all of them, especially the more corpulent among them. We have no way of knowing whether the citizens of Tarsus were particularly beefy, like the natives of some Pacific Islands, and if they were then perhaps they experienced sleep disordered breathing more than others, or perhaps Chrysostom used snoring as a parable for the citizens' carefree life of idleness. Whatever the reason, his oration was the first and possibly the only philosophical treatise on snoring.

H. V. Morton, a London journalist whose tales of his travels laid the foundations for a new style of tourist-journalist writing, despised snoring and snorers. From his travels in Ireland he recalls a nocturnal experience of sleeping with an extraordinary snorer who, without doubt, suffered from sleep apnea syndrome.

> Whenever I think of Kilkenny I shall remember the world's most accomplished snorer. I arrived late at night. The old castle of Kilkenny was lifted against the stars, with the dark river flowing against its walls, and, content with this glimpse of an ancient city, I went to bed dog-weary.
>
> I awakened in the middle of the night with the vague feeling that something unusual was happening. At first, because I was between sleeping and waking, I thought that a great sea was beating against the rocks, or it might have been the tramp of an army. This indecision lasted only for the fraction of a second, because I awakened to the sound of snoring so loud, so remarkable, so vibrant, so sure of itself that had it been produced consciously, it would have been the work of a genius.

I detest snorers. I regard snoring as a contemptible and disgraceful thing. I think that the woman married to a snorer should be granted a divorce without any argument. It has always seemed to me a singular reflection on modern science that no silencer has yet been invented for this complaint. During the war, when most of us slept in tents and tin huts, a boot, though primitive, was effective. But no boot could have interrupted the snorer of Kilkenny. He actually shook the air. He filled the universe. I could feel his bass notes in the wall.

How that man made me suffer. His ghastly organ recital was as regular in its devilish rhythm as a saw-mill. Once every half-hour he was seized with a kind of convulsion. I hoped that he was dying. The debasing sounds shuddered to pianissimo and ceased, then he gave a violent gasp, a snort, appeared to be choking, grunted, gasped, and got into top gear again.

Every man should be compelled to produce a certificate before marriage to prove that he is free from this horrible malady. I am glad, for the honour of Ireland, to say that he was an English commercial traveller. (H. V. Morton, *The Search for Ireland,* Methuen, London, 1930, pp. 66–67)

Morton awoke bleary-eyed in the morning and was unable to enjoy Kilkenny. But snoring is not only a matter for levity—there are those who discuss and study it with scientific gravity.

Snoring occurs as a result of vibration of the soft tissues in the area of the soft palate and pharynx due to the flow of air over them; it can be likened to the vibration of window-blind slats as the wind blows through them. The tendency to snore increases the narrower the airways are, and the more surplus tissue they have. We have seen that snoring does not occur in an environment of weightlessness, so it is easy to understand why it is so common among the obese and in situations in which the tonus of the smooth muscles is lax, such as when lying on the back or after drinking alcohol, and hence the expression "drunken snoring."

Although folklore draws no distinction between the various types of snoring or between one kind of snorer and another, modern research employs precise methods of measurement and assessment to classify

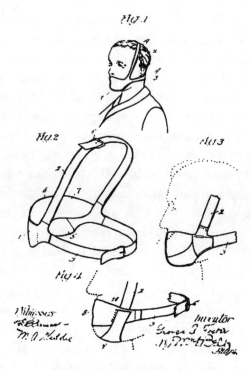

An antisnoring device that closes the
mouth, which was registered as a
U.S. patent in 1917

and quantify snoring. First, a distinction is made between chronic snorers, who snore every night in any position and situation, and those who
snore infrequently. These include people who snore only when they
sleep on their backs or after overindulging in alcoholic beverages. There
is a wide range of intermediate types between the two extremes, like
those who snore "twice or three times a week." The loudness of snoring,
too, is not uniform. Precise instruments, like those used to measure engine noise, show that snoring intensity can vary between twenty and
eighty decibels. As an illustration of what this means, the noise produced
by a motorcycle engine at full power is approximately eighty decibels.

Although almost every snore bears witness to the increased effort to
breathe during sleep, continuous and prolonged snoring does not usually
indicate the existence of sleep apnea syndrome. As mentioned earlier, the

snoring of people afflicted with sleep apnea syndrome is extraordinary in that it is not continuous, but interrupted. The most common pattern is a series of four to six increasingly loud snores that are replaced by total silence lasting for thirty to forty-five seconds, and so on. On numerous occasions I have heard from the spouse of a sleep apnea patient how she has been seized by panic on hearing her husband suddenly stop snoring. The tense wait for the renewal of the snoring, and the fear that its suspension will be permanent, drives sleep from the eyes of these patients' partners. Interrupted snoring is so characteristic of the syndrome that in extreme cases it can be diagnosed by listening to a recording of it.

The Touch of Morpheus

Since the early descriptions of Pickwickian patients first appeared in medical literature, excessive sleepiness has become the hallmark of the obese, rubicund person. Modern medical language does not leave much room for a description of the excessively sleepy person, and doctors' summaries are typically sparing in their use of words: "The patient tends to fall asleep in passive situations," or "The patient reports falling asleep while driving." In contrast, the language used by nineteenth-century physicians was far richer and more animated. One of the most colorful descriptions of an excessively sleepy patient appears in *The Philosophy of Sleep* by R. McNish, published in 1834. McNish, who accepted the fact that people sometimes complained of excessive sleepiness that was unrelated to a known illness, described the sleepy patient thus:

> The drowsy or sleepy persons have a disposition to sleep on every occasion. They do so at all times, and in all places. They sleep after dinner; they sleep in the theatre; they sleep in church. It is the same to them in what situation they may be placed: sleep is the great end of their existence—their occupation—their sole enjoyment. Morpheus is the deity at whose shrine they worship—the only god whose inference over them is omnipotent. . . . Let them sail, or ride, or sit, or lie, or walk, sleep overtakes them, binds their facilities in torpor. . . .

These are one dull, heavy-headed, drowsy mortals, those sons and daughters of phlegm—with passion as inert as a clutch-fog, and intellects as sluggish as the movements of the hypopotamus or leviathan. (p. 211)

Another piquant description of "the touch of Morpheus" (the god of dreams in Greek mythology) appears in the minutes of the New York Neurological Society from 1883 and comes from the testimony of a young doctor who suffered from excessive sleepiness.

I began the study of medicine, and it was during the lectures' hours that I was first troubled with my inability to keep awake. During the three years of my attendance upon medical lectures I do not think there was a single day when I did not at least once during the lectures either go soundly asleep or pass into a state of semiconsciousness. . . . This condition of things has grown steadily worse, until now I seldom can read more than half an hour—often not longer than fifteen minutes—without falling asleep. I would often, thinking it might only be a mental habit which could be broken by opposition, fight against this sleepiness for hours. . . . I have gone to sleep while making a vaginal examination in a case of labor. Three times during the writing of a single prescription I have nodded off in a momentary doze. I have gone to sleep in a dental chair while the pounding of gold filling was going on. (J. Morton, "A Case of Morbid Somnolence," *Journal of Nervous and Mental Diseases* 9 (1884): 617)

Although on the face of it these descriptions sound rather extreme, their translation into modern medical parlance fits patients who bear a severe form of sleep apnea. Not all the sufferers, however, are so sleepy, and complaints of excessive sleepiness vary in severity from patient to patient.

In mild cases the patient does not complain at all about a tendency to fall asleep during the day, but only about chronic tiredness that starts immediately after awakening from a night's sleep. Many patients define it something like this: "Doctor, when I wake up in the morning I'm more tired than I was before I went to sleep." This feeling of fatigue usually continues throughout the day and does not dissipate even after a long sleep such as one enjoys at weekends or on vacation. In slightly more severe cases the patient complains of a tendency to fall asleep, especially in passive, "sleep-inducing" situations like lectures, on long journeys, or while watching television or a movie. In particularly severe cases there is a tendency to fall asleep under any circumstances, during activities like eating, a telephone conversation, a social occasion, or even in such life-threatening situations as driving. These are the patients who fit Mc-Nish's description, and their story is similar to that of the sleepy New York doctor.

The questionnaires we use for diagnosing sleep disorders include a number of questions that try to establish the severity of the sleepiness. The subject is asked to indicate at what frequency he or she has fallen asleep during everyday activities such as reading, watching television, seeing a movie or play, while traveling as a passenger, during lectures, or at a social event. The subject can choose between "never," "infrequently," "often," and "always."

Even people who are aware of their tendency to fall asleep during the day will quite often deny it vehemently. I have seen this numerous times when couples visit our sleep laboratory for a consultation. While the woman complains that her husband embarrasses her by falling asleep on social occasions, the husband vigorously denies his wife's story, claiming that it is all in her mind.

So how can we determine, objectively and accurately, to what degree a specific person is sleepy during the day? Professor Mary Carskadon, head of the Brown University Sleep Laboratory and a student of William Dement, developed a simple and effective test to evaluate daily sleepiness levels. The test comprises five attempts, for half an hour each, to fall asleep under laboratory conditions, at 8 A.M., 10 A.M., noon, 4 P.M., and 6 P.M., and it is always conducted after a night's sleep of at least eight hours. Brain wave recordings determine the moment of falling asleep, which tells how long it took the subject to fall asleep, or sleep latency. Hence, it is called the multiple sleep latency test (MSLT). If the subject does not fall asleep within half an hour, he or she is moved from the bed-room to an adjoining room until the following attempt. People without sleep disorders find it hard to fall asleep during the day, even in a dark, soundproof room, and if they do succeed it happens only after twenty minutes or more. In contrast, those with sleep deprivation or pathologi-cal sleepiness will fall asleep during the day almost immediately after being told to do so. Sleep apnea syndrome patients fall asleep within ten minutes at every attempt, with an average time for sleep latency of five minutes or less. It should be emphasized that nothing changes in the daily sleepiness levels even if the subjects have slept for ten or twelve hours the night before the test.

The multiple sleep latency test can also help in diagnosing the causes of excessive sleeping, albeit not completely. If, for example, it is found that the subject who falls asleep quickly during the day goes di-rectly into REM sleep, this may be evidence of narcolepsy, especially if in addition to daytime sleepiness the subject complains of attacks of muscular weakness. On the other hand, a subject who complains of ex-cessive sleepiness but is unable to fall asleep in the daytime tests is al-most certainly suffering from chronic sleep deprivation, not necessarily from a sleep disorder, assuming that he or she slept for eight hours on the night before the test.

Restless Sleep

Anyone observing the sleep of a sleep apnea patient often sees a tempes-tuous scene. Every minute or two the patient's upper body rises with the help of the elbows, the chest heaves violently, and every muscle in the body strains in an effort to renew breathing. The effort ceases once the blockage in the airways is freed and is renewed with the next suspension of breathing. In most cases the patient is unaware of this nocturnal drama, but there are those who complain of frequent awakenings or of difficulty in falling asleep. These people are characterized by high sensi-tivity to external or internal stimuli during sleep, so they are conscious of some of their nocturnal awakenings. As the apneas and the awaken-ings appear immediately after falling asleep, they find it difficult to fall into continuous sleep and as a result also complain of difficulty in falling asleep in general. We have found that complaints of insomnia are more characteristic of adult sleep apnea patients, especially those over sixty, whose sleep is characterized by very little deep sleep. The high level of shallow sleep in older patients may explain why they are more aware of nocturnal awakenings than their younger counterparts.

"Doctor, I Wake Up with a Blinding Headache Every Morning!"

There is a long-running debate in the medical literature about whether the complaint of waking up with a "blinding headache" every morning is a symptom of sleep apnea syndrome. One-fifth of all severe sleep apnea sufferers in the various studies report that headaches on awakening were the reason for their coming to the sleep laboratory. However, our experience shows that complaints of headache on awakening are very common among people with a variety of sleep disorders and are not exclusive to sleep apnea syndrome. The incidence of complaints of headaches among sleep apnea syndrome patients is similar to that among all the people examined at sleep laboratories, with no relation to the test findings. Complaints of headaches that are not accompanied by complaints of snoring and sleepiness, therefore, should not be viewed as a clear symptom of sleep breathing disorders.

And What About Moods?

Although sleep apnea patients often complain of low spirits, irritability, or a reduced sexual drive, these complaints, too, are not exclusive to the syndrome. One can hear similar complaints from people with a wide range of sleep disorders, such as insomnia, narcolepsy, and restless legs syndrome, so they should not be viewed as a symptom of sleep breathing disorders unless accompanied by the characteristic complaints of snoring, daytime sleepiness, or evidence of apneas during sleep. But suspensions of breathing during sleep are indeed likely to cause sexual dysfunction in men, as we shall see later.

10

The Price of Awakenings

Anyone who has experienced a sleepless night does not need the scientific term "daytime sleepiness" explained. The greater the lack of sleep, the greater the struggle against drooping eyelids during the day. In this state, the need for sleep exceeds the need for food or drink.

Sleep apnea syndrome patients do not suffer from sleep deprivation. On the contrary, most patients claim that they get sufficient sleep and perhaps even sleep longer than healthy people, but they are unaware that they awaken every minute during the night. These awakenings are the price the brain pays to ensure resumption of breathing. The repeated disruptions in sleep continuity affect sleep structure, mainly by significantly reducing the amount of deep sleep and dream sleep. If we take into account that sleep apnea patients endure breathing disorders during sleep for several years before seeking treatment, we can understand why they walk around bleary-eyed during the day. Daytime sleepiness has a great impact on a person's quality of life and functional ability, and especially on the risk of being injured in accidents.

Several studies have employed a variety of tests to assess the ability of sleep apnea patients to function during the day. Most of the studies indicate that the syndrome is associated with a decline in intellectual abilities, which is hardly surprising. A sleepy person will find it difficult to perform tasks that require concentration and focused attention, especially when the tasks are prolonged and monotonous, and will have less difficulty performing short, interesting tasks. Similar findings have been reported on people who have been deprived of sleep for extended periods.

So it is not hard to deduce that the functioning of sleep apnea patients is impaired. Naturally, a decline in functional ability has considerable significance for professional advancement, income, and satisfaction with one's work environment and conditions. In the study of industrial workers described earlier, we found that complaints of sleep disorders were strongly associated with a number of factors related to the work environment. Workers who complained of daytime sleepiness were less satisfied with their work than others; they also were involved in more work-related accidents or close calls, tended toward more frequent absenteeism, and reported tension with colleagues and supervisors.

But it is not only the patient's quality of life at work that is impaired. The term "quality of life" encompasses a variety of factors associated with a person's ability to function at work, at home, within the narrow family circle and the wider social one, as well as personal feelings and expectations regarding physical and mental health, and a belief that personal goals and dreams are being achieved. In recent years several questionnaires have been designed to quantify all this with a measurement of "quality of life." The study of Wisconsin civil servants by Young and her colleagues used a detailed questionnaire to evaluate quality of life, and it was found that people with sleep apnea had "poorer quality of life" than those who were untouched by the syndrome. People with the syndrome complained of limited ability to function caused by physical problems, impaired social functioning, and a general decline in their feeling of health. The same people also reported insufficient energy to deal with upkeep of their homes or even recreation, as well as social isolation. Furthermore, they seldom read due to a low falling-asleep threshold, which gave rise to frustration and even a sense of anxiety and helplessness. It is sometimes difficult to distinguish between the direct influence of sleep disorders and the influence of illnesses accompanying the syndrome. But successful treatment of the syndrome improved these patients' scores on the quality of life index, which by itself shows that sleep breathing disorders have a measurable impact on quality of life.

And What About Your Sex Life?

Sex life is a central factor in quality of life, although very few studies have specifically addressed this issue in sleep apnea patients. A possible association between a decline in sexual function and sleep apnea was found during examinations of penile erections during sleep carried out to identify causes of impotency. Among its other physiological characteristics, REM sleep in men tends to be accompanied by a full or partial erection. Although there is still no adequate explanation for why nocturnal erections occur, they have considerable clinical implications. Since nocturnal erections occur regardless of dream content or sexual activity before sleep, recording them may provide information on the functioning of the penile erection mechanism. Impotency can be the result of mental or organic causes. When the cause is mental, the erection mechanism remains functional during sleep. When the cause is organic, nocturnal erections do not occur.

Ismet Karacan, a psychiatrist and veteran sleep researcher born in Istanbul, was one of the first to use the "nocturnal erection test" to conduct a differential diagnosis to distinguish between mental and organic problems. To his surprise, he found in men who had been examined following complaints of impotency that a relatively large number also suffered from breathing disorders during sleep. Moreover, in some of the men there was an improvement in sexual function when the sleep breathing disorders were successfully treated. Since we drew similar conclusions from nocturnal erection tests at the Technion's sleep laboratory, we decided to examine the sexual activity and enjoyment of sex life among sleep apnea patients.

We randomly selected two hundred patients from those who had been examined at our laboratory and interviewed them about their sex lives. We found that the severity of sleep disordered breathing was directly correlated with less sexual activity and enjoyment of sex life. Complaints of diminishing sexual activity were not secondary to complaints of daytime fatigue and sleepiness, but depended on the severity of apneas and on the degree of falling saturation levels in blood oxygen. To investigate the reasons for patients' impaired sex lives, we collaborated with Rafael Luboshitzky, head of the endocrinology institute at HaEmek Hospital in Afula, in a study of testosterone levels during sleep, comparing sleep apnea patients with a control group that didn't have breathing disorders. Daily testosterone secretion rates, which in healthy men peak during sleep, were considerably lower in sleep apnea patients than in the control group. In half the patients testosterone levels were so low that the hormone would have to be administered artificially before they would be able to resume a normal sex life. When the patients were examined again three months after commencing treatment for the syndrome, we found a significant increase in their testosterone secretion.

These findings indicate that at least some of the reasons for diminished libido and enjoyment of sex life among sleep apnea patients are associated with suppressed secretion of the male sex hormone caused by apneas, or as a result of disrupted sleep. Effective treatment of the syndrome may improve secretion of the hormone and patients' sex lives. To date, no information is available on the possibility of similar changes occurring in women's sexual activity and quality of sex life, and whether secretion of the sex hormones is suppressed in women too.

Falling Asleep at the Wheel—Chronicle of an Accident Foretold

The greatest price of nightly disruptions in sleep is the risk of accidents, especially traffic accidents. Almost falling asleep at the wheel is not uncommon: surveys in various countries show that at least one in every three drivers has had this experience at least once. When it happens, there is a gradual restriction of the driver's field of vision, and a detachment from the road and his or her surroundings. These sensations are accompanied by an almost uncontrollable desire to close one's eyes "just for a couple of seconds." Very few people, however, admit to stopping their vehicle on the roadside for a brief nap or to stretch their legs to relieve sleepiness. The urge to continue driving despite acute feelings of sleepiness is rooted in a firm belief that "it won't happen to me," which outweighs any fears of a possible accident.

People with no sleep disorders have daytime sleepiness crises too, but they generally overcome them within forty to forty-five minutes. Quite naturally, wakefulness levels are not constant throughout the day, and sleepiness crises tend to be replaced every one and a half to two hours by periods of heightened alertness. This is not the case in people who are affected by sleep deficiency or chronic disruptions in their sleep. They are sleepy throughout the whole day, from the moment they open their eyes upon awakening until they go to sleep at night.

A few years ago, on a heavily laden bus hurtling down the Jerusalem–Tel Aviv expressway, I witnessed a driver falling asleep that demonstrated graphically how dangerous people can be in this state, both to themselves and to others. Immediately upon leaving Jerusalem, the passenger next to me drew my attention to the bus driver's face reflected in the mirror above his head. It did not require a sleep research specialist to see that the driver was on the verge of falling asleep. He was yawning incessantly, his eyes were half closed, and his eyelids occasionally fell completely shut. We were not the only ones who noticed his condition. A young soldier sitting in the seat next to the driver got out of her seat, took a bottle of water from her bag, and asked him politely but firmly to stop at the roadside and splash some water on his face, which he did. By this point all the passengers had become aware of his condition, and they kept an anxious eye on his driving.

Splashing water on his face helped for only a few minutes. As the journey progressed, the driver's head started swinging from side to side, and the bus swerved dangerously out of its lane and off the road several times. That was when I decided that fate had been sufficiently tempted. I got out of my seat and told the driver that if he did not stop at the side of the road the passengers would sue him and the company for reckless driving. Happily, no further persuasion was required. The driver stopped, and we waited patiently until a more alert substitute arrived. I do not know why the driver was so sleepy. Perhaps he didn't get enough sleep the previous night, perhaps he had severe sleep disorders, maybe even sleep apnea, but his insistence on continuing to drive despite his sleepiness was more than enough evidence that he did not make the connection between his condition and safety when driving. Unfortunately, he is not alone in this, as has been shown by researchers in several countries.

The first study on falling asleep while driving, which became a classic, was conducted by Torbjorn Akerstedt of the Karolinska Institute in Stockholm in 1987. Akerstedt recorded the brain waves of train drivers working night shifts on the Nassjo–Stockholm route, a distance of some 240 kilometers. Analysis of the recordings showed that along extensive sections of the track, the brain waves indicated that about a quarter of the drivers experienced episodes of sleepiness and sometimes even fell asleep. In one instance the driver missed a signal to reduce his speed from 130 kilometers per hour to 90, which could have easily ended in disaster.

About ten years later, Merrill Mitler and his colleagues from a sleep laboratory in San Diego installed video cameras in the driver's cabs of several of the huge rigs that hurtle across the United States and Canada every day. The cameras recorded the drivers' faces during their journeys; some drivers also had their brain waves recorded. The results of this study were alarming: the video recordings showed that several drivers spent a large part of their journey in a state of acute sleepiness, occasionally even experiencing brief episodes of sleep, particularly during nighttime driving. These findings were not unusual, however. Interviews with 593 truck drivers in the United States, randomly selected at rest stops and filling stations, showed that almost half admitted to falling asleep while driving at least once in their lives. A quarter of them admitted that they had fallen asleep while driving in the previous year.

In Israel, according to official statistics kept by the police, only 1 percent of all road accidents are classified as "sleep accidents." This assertion is not unequivocal and is based on circumstantial evidence. When dealing with a driver only, classification of an accident as sleep-related is based on suspicious findings, such as unexplained swerving from a straight road and no signs of braking. Classification of an accident is much easier when there are witnesses to it. Although the number of sleep-related traffic accidents is relatively small compared with the vast number of all traffic accidents in Israel, their outcomes are particularly serious. The number of fatalities caused by sleep-related accidents is four to five times that of accidents from other causes. But sleep accidents are just the tip of the iceberg. Road safety experts are convinced that 30 to 40 percent of accidents are caused by a drop in the driver's level of alertness. At a speed of 100 kilometers per hour, even a momentary loss of concentration is sufficient for a vehicle to deviate from its course and crash into a tree or an oncoming vehicle. We don't have accurate data on the percentage of accidents caused by fatigue or sleepiness, but it can be safely assumed that the figure is high, especially in accidents caused by swerving off course, which usually result in injuries and fatalities.

Because sleep apnea syndrome is the most prevalent cause of day-time sleepiness, especially in men, it is hardly surprising that almost a hundred scientific papers have been published in several languages on the involvement of sleep apnea patients in road accidents. There are but few instances in which agreement among researchers is so extensive as it is on the association between sleep apnea and accidents.

Antonio Jimenez and his colleagues examined the sleep of 102 drivers who had received medical treatment following traffic accidents. Their subjects were selected from patients at two hospitals in northern Spain, one at either end of a particular stretch of expressway between Santander and Burgos. The researchers compared their findings on these drivers with those from 152 randomly sampled people of the same ages and genders. The prevalence of sleep apnea syndrome was six times higher in the group of drivers who had been injured in accidents than in the control group. The results of the study were published in the *New England Journal of Medicine,* and it had great practical impact on drivers with sleep apnea in Spain. Following the study, driving regulations were amended to prohibit sleep apnea patients from driving unless they were being treated for the condition.

Simulated studies assessing the driving abilities of sleep apnea patients have also shown that they are prone to accidents. John Stradling's group from Oxford, England, demonstrated that sleep apnea patients assessed with a simulator had difficulty staying in their lane and noticing changes along the route, especially in limited visibility conditions. Effective treatment of the syndrome improved patients' driving performance. David Dinges from Philadelphia, one of the top experts worldwide on the effect of sleep deficiency on cognitive and psychomotor performance, showed that the decline in driving abilities of sleep apnea patients depends on the amount of time they spend driving: these patients had difficulty driving continuously for longer than thirty minutes.

The issue gains in importance when coupled with evidence that the prevalence of sleep apnea syndrome in professional drivers is higher than in the general population. The sleep laboratory in Stanford conducted sleep recordings on 150 randomly selected truck drivers. Considerable sleep disordered breathing, of more than thirty apneas per hour, was found in 10 percent of the drivers. The drivers with sleep disordered breathing were overweight and also tended to suffer from hypertension. It is frightening to imagine the consequences if 10 percent of all the truck drivers on the highways are operating with such a grave disability.

In response to such fears, committees of the American Medical Association and various European medical organizations have grappled long and hard with what to do about sleep apnea patients and driving, and even whether they should have their driver's licenses suspended. Doctors are expected to consider the public's best interest as well as those of their patients, but patients also have a right to privacy and doctor-patient confidentiality. Furthermore, practical considerations cannot be ignored. Patients who know that their doctors are supposed to report to the authorities that they are not competent to drive may try to conceal the disability. Even without suspecting doctors' intentions, many sleep apnea patients tend to deny their sleepiness.

A European task force published its conclusions on the subject in 1999, and the scientific council of the American Medical Association issued a report in 1998. Both, however, avoided recommending that sleep apnea patients' licenses be revoked. The Europeans called for a distinction between drivers of private vehicles and drivers of public vehicles, and they recommended implementing stricter restrictions on professional drivers. The Americans issued only a general recommendation to heighten awareness of the association between sleepiness and traffic accidents, especially among professional drivers.

Whether these organizations ever decide to take a firm position on the subject of apnea patients and driving, and whether any other societies will follow the lead of Spain in doing something about it, it is clear that the consequences of sleep disorders are great. People with sleep apnea syndrome are not just subject to dozing during the day: it detracts from their enjoyment of their work and of their life in general, particularly their sex life. They are also a danger to those around them, especially when they get behind the wheel of a car. As if that weren't enough, apneas can also directly threaten people's lives, especially certain babies and people with cardiac conditions, as we shall see once we find out more about some related sleep disorders.

11

At the Temple of Morpheus

Diagnosing sleep apnea syndrome has become the principal occupation of experts and doctors who treat sleep disorders. The vast majority of sleep laboratory examinees seek advice because of suspected sleep apnea, and in many hospitals, particularly in departments treating pulmonary and ear, nose, and throat illnesses, recent years have seen the establishment of sleep laboratories for diagnosing the syndrome. The term "sleep apnea syndrome" has in fact replaced "narcolepsy" as a synonym for chronic sleepiness.

But a day-to-day preoccupation with only one syndrome, prevalent though it might be, is liable to conceal the fact that excessive sleepiness may derive from other sleep disorders, as the following case graphically shows. Some years ago, a psychiatrist friend referred a young woman to me for a consultation. She was a nurse who worked in my friend's hospital department, and she had been complaining for a long time of tiredness and low spirits. Her tiredness and her large physical dimensions made it easy to suspect sleep apnea syndrome. Indeed she was very fat, with a short thick neck, and she told me that she felt a tremendous desire to sleep during the day, which was causing her great hardship in both her work and her private life. During the interview, I told her that the cause of her complaints was almost certainly treatable and that all she needed was a sleep test to verify the diagnosis.

To my chagrin, however, the test findings refuted my preliminary diagnosis. Her breathing was completely normal and regular throughout the course of sleep. The only finding that deviated from the norm, in fact, was her dream sleep latency—the duration of time that elapses from the moment of falling asleep to the appearance of the first dream period. In people with no sleep disorders or other illnesses, this period is about an hour and a half, whereas our nurse started dreaming after about half that time—in approximately forty minutes. Short dream sleep latency is typical of narcoleptic or depressive patients. But her complaints were inconsistent with narcolepsy, and I found the possibility of depression odd because she was a psychiatric nurse who had been referred by a psychiatrist who knew her well. I assumed that, had she been suffering from depression, the problem would have been diagnosed before she had come to see me. So I asked her to come in for another visit.

At the second meeting, she began by telling me that she had slept through the laboratory examination "just like I sleep at home," and that she hoped the examination had helped in diagnosing her sleep disorder. I asked her if she had noticed any change in her mood since she began feeling the strong urge to sleep—whereupon, to my great surprise, her eyes filled with tears that rolled uncontrollably down her cheeks. After she had collected herself, she told me that for some months she had been feeling a deep depression, which caused her great panic because her mother had suffered from severe depression and had even tried to take her own life. Because of her training as a psychiatric nurse, she was aware of the possibility that she had inherited the illness from her mother, and this was why she had repressed the thought of her own depression—so much so that all that remained was a strong need to sleep. Her constant preoccupation with tiredness had successfully taken over from her troublesome thoughts about depression. In the wake of this revelation, she began a course of anti-depressant medication that greatly enhanced her mood and reduced her degree of tiredness.

The lesson to be learned is clear. There must be no rush to diagnose sleep apnea syndrome on the basis of first impressions given by complaints of sleepiness, even when they come from a very obese patient—or even from an obese and sleepy patient who also complains of loud snoring. Other disorders, too, may be manifested in a similar way.

Narcolepsy

At the end of the nineteenth century and in the first half of the twentieth, anyone afflicted with excessive sleepiness was almost automatically categorized as narcoleptic. "Narcolepsy" refers to a defined syndrome with clear and characteristic symptoms, a syndrome that is fortunately rare, especially in Israel—but more about that later.

The narcoleptic patient experiences uncontrollable attacks of falling asleep during the day, and these can occur under almost any circumstances, including extremely embarrassing ones such as while eating, during a telephone conversation, or even while driving. The patient is also subjected to severe muscular laxity that causes him or her to fall. This combination of muscular laxity and sleeping attacks gave rise in the past to the suspicion that narcolepsy might be a form of epilepsy, and this was the basis of the erroneous theory regarding the illness that found its way into several medical books. Unlike healthy people or those with sleep disorders and attacks of excessive sleepiness, especially under conditions of inactivity, in narcoleptic patients the circumstances surrounding attacks of sleepiness and muscular laxity are truly extraordinary—for they appear when the patient gets excited. These attacks can manifest themselves during outbursts of anger, joy, laughter, weeping, or even when the patient is surprised. It is entirely possible that the expressions "my knees were knocking" and "he was paralyzed with terror," which describe physical reactions to situations of extreme excitement, also express the relationship between emotional excitement and the attacks of muscular weakness suffered by narcoleptics.

One of the first narcoleptics to be examined at the Technion Sleep Laboratory in Haifa said that the most annoying thing of all was that his attacks of "paralysis," as he described them, always occurred when his grandchildren came to visit. Another patient, who was a teacher, said that she didn't dare raise her voice at her pupils because even the smallest loss of temper would bring on an attack. Much to her chagrin, her pupils exploited this to the full! Two additional symptoms characterize some narcoleptics. One of these is hypnagogic hallucinations, which usually appear during the falling-asleep process and take the form of clear and detailed dreams that are often mixed with the last sights and sounds the patient saw and heard before the attack. One of our patients was afflicted with uncontrollable sleep during bus journeys, and she told us that the attacks were always accompanied by dreams in bright green; only years later did she realize that this was also the color of the seats on the bus. The other characteristic symptom is paralysis on awakening. A patient who awakens from an attack of narcolepsy experiences a feeling of acute paralysis that can last for a number of seconds, or even minutes, which causes a deep sense of panic because the patient feels that he or she is not breathing and is liable to suffocate.

The first to put a name to this illness was the French physician Jean-Baptiste-Edouard Gelineau. In 1880, he saw in his clinic a Parisian wine-barrel merchant who complained of attacks of falling asleep at any time, as often as two hundred times a day! The attacks might occur during physical effort, when he was emotionally excited, or even when he was sexually aroused. The merchant, who had a healthy sense of humor, found it difficult to go to the theater, according to Gelineau, for every laugh would bring on an immediate sleeping attack. He also experienced great muscular weakness during his attacks, which on more than one occasion had caused him to fall down like a drunk. Gelineau took great pains to point out that the collapse of the narcoleptic was caused by sleep, whereas in an epileptic attack sleep followed the patient's collapse. Despite this sharp distinction made by Gelineau, narcolepsy and epilepsy were confused for many years, and this confusion found its way into medical literature.

Ever since Gelineau first described narcolepsy, an overabundance of assumptions has accumulated regarding its source. At the beginning of the twentieth century the illness was widely thought to be a mental reaction to stress and frustration. Some viewed it as a defense mechanism against latent aggression, or even excessive sexuality; patients presumably escaped into sleep because they were unable to cope with their sex drives. This assumption was reinforced by the fact that the symptoms of narcolepsy first appear in adolescence, and accordingly narcoleptics were given psychological treatment.

The first real breakthrough occurred with the earliest sleep recordings of narcoleptic patients. Only then did it become clear that the structure of narcoleptics' sleep is vastly different from that of other people. Sleep in most people begins with sleep stages other than REM sleep, and they reach the first REM cycle only after ninety minutes or so. But the sleep rhythm of narcoleptics is reversed; they fall directly into REM sleep. This reversal exists in sleep that takes place both at night and during the day. This finding fully explained the strange characteristics of narcoleptic sleep attacks. REM sleep, as we know, is characterized by both muscle paralysis and dreams. In other words, the muscle laxity that narcoleptics experience during an attack of sleep and the lucid dreams they report at the conclusion of their attack are both part of normal REM sleep. In contrast to most people, who remain unaware of events that occur during REM sleep unless they awaken in the middle of it, narcoleptics who fall directly into REM sleep during their daily routine cannot fail to be aware of them.

Narcoleptic Dogs

Impressive progress has been made over the past fifteen years in understanding the source of narcolepsy. Solving the riddle was somewhat similar to completing a jigsaw puzzle, with another missing piece being discovered every few years, until the entire picture became clear in 2000. Narcolepsy has always been difficult to understand, and it only became more so in 1984, when Professor Yukata Honda of Seiwa Hospital in Tokyo surprised narcolepsy researchers with his discovery of a common factor in the blood of 135 Japanese narcoleptics. In all of them, the immune system used a molecule known as DR2 for identifying the body's cells. In the immune system, human leukocyte antigens (HLA) are used to distinguish between "friendly" and "enemy" cells, so that the immune system attacks invaders and not the body's healthy cells. Certain molecules adhere to the body's cells and fly a "marker" that the immune system's cells recognize, so that they then attack only foreign cells or cells whose protein production mechanism has malfunctioned due to the incursion of viruses. Genetic markers are of vital practical importance in organ transplants because a patient can be given an organ from another person only if both their immune systems use the same molecules for identifying the body's cells. When the identification system does not work properly, the immune system is liable to attack healthy cells, as in those illnesses known as autoimmune diseases.

The relationship between the HLA system and narcolepsy was found not only in Japanese patients but also in other ethnic groups. It seems that 95 percent of all narcoleptics carry the same marker of the HLA system. This, however, was later identified not as DR2 but as a DQ1 molecule. At first these findings led to the assumption that narcolepsy is a genetic illness, but it quickly became clear that this was not so. First, although the risk of a narcoleptic's relatives falling victim to the illness is approximately ten times higher than in the general population, the number of family cases is relatively small. Moreover, even in identical twins the illness has been found in both siblings in only 25–30 percent of the cases. But when it seemed that narcolepsy research had reached a blind alley there was another breakthrough, this time from a totally unexpected direction.

In contrast to sleep apnea syndrome, which is exclusive to human beings, narcolepsy is not. It became clear in the 1970s that there are also narcoleptic dogs, especially in the golden retriever and Doberman breeds. Narcoleptic dogs are sleepy during the day and suffer muscular weakness attacks when excited, just like humans. For two decades now, Bill Dement has been raising a group of narcoleptic dogs at the Stanford Sleep Disorders and Research Center, and they have played a central role in solving the riddle. In dogs, unlike in humans, narcolepsy is hereditary, and—as though made to order for the researchers—the hereditary form in dogs is relatively simple. Narcolepsy in dogs is caused by a single recessive gene, which means the dog must receive the flawed gene from both parents for it to inherit the illness. In addition, all the offspring of a pair of narcoleptic dogs will also be narcoleptic. This fact enabled Dement and his team to raise several generations of narcoleptic dogs for the purposes of research.

Emmanuel Mignot is another French researcher who followed Christian Guilleminault to the Stanford University sleep laboratory. On his arrival, he set himself a single objective—to discover the gene that caused narcolepsy in dogs. Talent, diligence, sophisticated technology, and no small measure of intuition and luck are inherent in the race to identify genes, and Mignot and his team were blessed with an abundance of all. In August 1999, ten years after they embarked on their project, they reported in the scientific journal *Cell* on the identification of the gene responsible for narcolepsy in dogs. The gene, found on chromosome 12 of the dog, is responsible for producing a protein that serves as a receptor for another protein called hypocretin. This protein is secreted by a small group of cells located in the hypothalamus, a minuscule region deep in the brain that controls hunger, thirst, sexual activity, and sleep. Hypocretin connects with special receptors, which as mentioned earlier are produced under the supervision of a single gene, and which are spread over cells in various locations in the brain, thus transmitting information to the target cell on how to act. The flawed gene in narcoleptic dogs caused the receptor not to connect with the hypocretin, thus blocking the flow of information from the cells producing the protein to the target cells.

What, then, is hypocretin's role and what information does it transmit to the target cells? Some two years before the identification of the narcolepsy gene, the protein, which is made up of thirty-three amino acids, was identified. It was initially found to be related to the regulation of eating, and its injection into rats' brain cells made them become ravenously hungry—hence the protein's other name, orexin. Immediately afterward it was also found that hypocretin plays an important role in the supervision of wakefulness levels and sleep rhythms. Proof of this also appeared in the issue of *Cell* in which Mignot's article was published. In order to examine how removal of the protein would affect the eating behavior of mice, Masashi Yanagisawa and his colleagues at the University of Texas in Dallas genetically produced mice lacking the hypocretin protein.

At first there was great disappointment, for it appeared that nothing had happened. The mice without hypocretin behaved exactly like their brothers that had the protein. But during the night, when mice are usually very energetic and active, the team discovered a strange phenomenon: the hypocretin-less mice were attacked every now and then, for a period of between thirty seconds and one minute, by what appeared to

Yanagisawa and his colleagues to be motoric paralysis. A mouse that had been running around its cage restlessly suddenly froze for about half a minute, and then continued running around as if nothing had happened. At first the team thought that the mice had undergone epileptic attacks, but the brain wave and muscle tonus recordings during these strange attacks contradicted this possibility. The researchers therefore concluded that the mice had suffered attacks of paralysis similar to those in narcoleptic humans and dogs. As the REM sleep of mice is very brief, from half a minute to a minute every now and again, so were the attacks of paralysis extremely short. The sleep recordings of hypocretin-less mice later showed disorders in their sleep patterns and a very rapid entry into REM sleep, exactly the same as had been found in narcoleptic humans and dogs.

It is quite amazing how two studies that were undertaken for totally different reasons—one searching for the flawed gene that causes narcolepsy, and the other studying the role of hypocretin in eating behavior—led to the same conclusions on the relationship between the protein and narcolepsy.

But is there any proof of a flaw in the production of hypocretin or in the hypocretin receptor in human narcoleptics? We now come to the last piece of the jigsaw that completed the picture. It became clear that the problem in humans was not a flaw in the formation of the protein receptor, but a dysfunction in the protein's production itself.

First, Mignot and his colleagues reported that no trace of hypocretin was found in the cerebral-spinal fluid in seven out of nine narcoleptics, while the protein was found in the spinal fluid of every one of the control group's subjects. The reason for this came to light immediately afterward. At the same time as the article appeared in *Cell,* Mignot and Jerry Siegel's group from the University of California in Los Angeles reported that, in the brains of narcoleptic patients who had died, they found no traces of the hypocretin-producing nerve cells in the hypothalamus. The researchers' assumption was that either these cells had not even been formed in the narcoleptics' brains or they had disappeared at a specific stage of development. In any event, this finding explained the fact that the protein could not be identified in the spinal fluid of narcoleptic patients, and it also provided solid proof that hypocretin plays a key role in the control of sleep and wakefulness.

What can be learned of the source of narcolepsy from the findings of recent years? It is currently assumed that narcolepsy may be an autoimmune illness in which the immune system attacks and destroys the group of hypocretin-producing cells in the hypothalamus. It is further assumed that the factor responsible for the appearance of the illness is environmental and, for a still-unknown reason, people susceptible to it carry the DQ1 genetic marker. It is very likely that the destruction of the cells takes place at an early age, and therefore its traces cannot be identified later. Following the destruction of the cells, a hypocretin deficiency is created, and as a result the messenger from the hypothalamus carrying the order "stay awake" does not reach the cells whose job it is to ensure wakefulness.

The relationship between narcolepsy and genetic markers has solved one of the riddles that puzzled me most regarding sleep disorders. Based on experience acquired in sleep laboratories all over the world, when I established Israel's first clinical sleep laboratory I was convinced that the majority of people seeking counseling for excessive sleepiness would turn out to be narcoleptics. Although the exact incidence of the illness in the general population is unknown, estimates suggest that it is one patient in every thousand people. This would mean we could expect to find at least one hundred thousand narcoleptics in Israel. As the illness limits the normal functioning of the patient to such a great extent, it was also reasonable to assume that narcoleptics would be diagnosed either at their army induction physical or during their military service. To my great surprise, the number of narcoleptics who came to the sleep laboratory was minimal—no more than ten patients in more than twenty-five years—during which time we saw some fifty thousand patients! There was a possibility that narcoleptic patients were being treated elsewhere and therefore had no need of the sleep laboratory, but we conducted a survey of every neurologist in the country and found that practically no new patients had joined the ranks of the ones we already knew about. According to our findings, there are only some twenty to thirty narcoleptics in Israel—a hundred times fewer than we had expected from data about other countries. As there are big differences in the prevalence of certain diseases and illnesses among various ethnic groups, one possibility was that narcolepsy is not a "Jewish" illness.

To examine this "Jewish question," I contacted a number of sleep researchers who worked in areas of the United States with large Jewish populations and asked them if they knew of any Jewish narcoleptics. Initially, they were somewhat insulted by the question: did I think that they pried into their patients' religious beliefs? Once I had placated them and explained why the information was so vital, I found that even doctors at the Montefiore Hospital Sleep Laboratory in New York, in the heart of the largest Jewish population in the United States, had difficulty remembering a single case of narcolepsy in a Jewish patient. These findings were repeated in numerous other locations.

The relationship between the HLA molecular marker and narcolepsy provided a partial answer to the riddle of why there are so few Jewish narcoleptics. It appears that there is a big difference between various ethnic groups in the prevalence of the gene that codes for the DQ1 molecule, which carries the complicated symbol DQB1*0602. While in Europe and the United States some 20–22 percent of the population are carriers, only 5–8 percent of Israelis carry it.

The genetic marker for narcolepsy is very prevalent in Japan. It is found in the blood of one in three Japanese, so it is hardly surprising that it was in Japan that the genetic marker in the blood of narcoleptics was first discovered, and that country has the highest number of narcoleptics in the world. If individuals carrying this genetic marker are indeed at particularly high risk of succumbing to narcolepsy, then this can explain the low incidence of the illness in Israel.

Narcolepsy is treated with stimulants that prevent the onset of the attacks of sleepiness, and these particular drugs must be used under the supervision of a doctor. The attacks of muscle paralysis are treated with drugs that prevent entry into REM sleep. Yet the new discoveries regarding the role of hypocretin promise the future development of new drugs for the exclusive treatment of narcolepsy.

Periodic Leg Movements During Sleep

One of the characteristics of sleep is the absence of motoric activity. Normally the only reason we move our limbs during sleep is to change position, and these movements characterize the transition from deep to light sleep and the entry into and exit from REM sleep. The number of gross body movements per night is constant and does not exceed twenty-five. But there are people whose sleep features excessive activity of the motoric system, especially movement of the lower limbs, or restless legs syndrome. These people move their legs during sleep in periodic movements every twenty seconds or so, in most cases both legs simultaneously, although these movements can be seen in only one leg or in both legs alternately. In addition, the range or size of the movement varies from person to person; in some they may involve the entire leg, as if the person is walking while lying down, while in others the movement may be small, involving only the big toe, for example. In severe cases the number of leg movements per night can reach somewhere between four hundred and five hundred, severely impairing the continuity of sleep. A great many of these leg movements cause a brief awakening, manifested by the appearance of alpha brain waves, accelerated heart rate, and increased blood pressure. The brain wakefulness level of people who move their legs excessively during sleep is high, so their sleep is not "effective." When these people awaken they feel great tiredness and tend to fall asleep in passive situations during the day.

It should be emphasized, however, that the most notable complaint of people with this syndrome is not necessarily sleepiness or daytime tiredness. Sometimes they are aware of their awakenings and will therefore complain of insomnia, difficulty in falling asleep, or difficulties in maintaining sleep continuity. The syndrome is easy to diagnose when the patients categorically complain of "restless legs," that their legs bother them when they are lying down and trying to sleep. Most people who complain of this problem are suffering from periodic leg movements. The discomfort in their legs is manifested in stiffness or "pins and needles" that are relieved only when they move around. The phenomenon of restless legs is called the Ekbom syndrome, after the physician who first described it in 1945, and it is common among people who have kidney disease and are undergoing dialysis, cardiac insufficiency, or Parkinson's disease, and also in the aged. Periodic leg movements during sleep can be treated with medication. When the leg movements during sleep disappear, so do the daytime sleepiness and insomnia.

The fact that periodic leg movements also appear in people who are paralyzed as a result of spinal column damage hints that the source of the movements is the motor cells in the spinal column that affect the legs without the brain's active participation. Although there are sleep apnea patients who move their legs during sleep, periodic leg movements frequently appear following effective treatment of the syndrome. There is still no proven explanation of this phenomenon, but it may explain why certain patients continue to complain of excessive tiredness despite the disappearance of their apneas during sleep.

Kleine-Levin Syndrome

Very few sleep experts have encountered people suffering from Kleine-Levin syndrome, which is a rare and exotic sleep disorder. Only some 150 patients with the syndrome have been described in the medical literature to date, 40 of whom were diagnosed at our laboratory—perhaps as compensation for the paucity of narcoleptics in Israel.

Sleep disorders in Kleine-Levin syndrome first appear during adolescence (around fifteen to sixteen years of age), and particularly among boys. In contrast to the daytime sleepiness of sleep apnea syndrome patients or the compulsive attacks of sleep in narcoleptics, Kleine-Levin syndrome patients have prolonged attacks of sleepiness that can continue for some ten days, when between the attacks their wakefulness is completely normal. These attacks of sleep are quite understandably a source of panic to adolescents' parents. Without warning, their alert, active son spends all his time asleep or half asleep, and if they do not force him to he neither eats nor drinks until the attack is over. The attack is not only manifested in a change in the level of wakefulness, for the entry into and exit from the attack of sleepiness can bring with them behavioral disturbances, some of which can be extremely embarrassing. Not only does the wakeful patient sink into a stupor for several days, but he may suddenly display an uncontrollable appetite and shameless sexual behavior. He has an uncontrollable urge to eat special foodstuffs like jelly or chocolate and can dispose of huge quantities of food in a very short time. Especially dramatic is the sexual coarseness of his behavior. One frightened mother told me that during an attack her son would undress in front of strangers visiting their home and publicly masturbate. She said that when the attack was over, this phenomenon passed as if it had never happened and her son refused to believe that he had behaved in a such a manner. Our experience shows that half of the patients suffer from eating and sexual behavior disorders that turn the attacks of sleep into traumatic events for the whole family.

The patients' medical history does not indicate an illness or injury that might explain the syndrome's appearance, but in many people the first attack appears close to an illness that is accompanied by a high fever or after a great physical or mental effort. In contrast to the attacks of sleep in narcolepsy or sleep apnea that can be controlled with stimulants, the majority of Kleine-Levin patients do not respond to medication. In cases like this, when medication is not efficacious, all that can be done is to assure the parents that their child's condition will return to normal at the end of the attack. In a follow-up study we conducted on more than thirty people with Kleine-Levin syndrome we found that the attacks waned with age in almost all of them. When they reached age twenty-five the sleep attacks were replaced by short attacks of tiredness and brief states of being half asleep. Once the patients passed thirty these, too, disappeared without trace.

We have no clear idea of the causes of Kleine-Levin syndrome, but the combination of attacks of sleep, uncontrollable hunger, and sexual drive all point to the hypothalamus. As mentioned earlier, the hypothalamus is a tiny portion of the brain—about the size of a small olive—that is linked to control of sleep and wakefulness and such drives as eating and sex, and is also connected to the production of hypocretin. Although we do not have imaging techniques that help us discern possible damage to the hypothalamus, its involvement in the secretion of various hormones provides an indirect means of examining its normal functioning. Disruptions in the secretion of hormones linked to the hypothalamus are indeed found in Kleine-Levin patients, supporting the suspicion of hypothalamus involvement in the syndrome. In light of the findings on the absence of hypothalamic cells that produce hypocretin in narcoleptics, it would be interesting to examine whether a disruption in the production of this protein is also linked to Kleine-Levin syndrome. So far, however, studies have not shown abnormalities in hypocretin levels in Kleine-Levin patients.

Idiopathic Excessive Sleep

The term "idiopathic" is generally used when we are at a loss to explain the source of a phenomenon. Some people are "naturally sleepy" and have no difficulty falling asleep anywhere and under any conditions—on the contrary, they have a big problem staying awake in monotonous circumstances. Most of them do not even complain about it, unless they are forced to stay awake for long periods. A "dozy" soldier, for instance, has real difficulty in staying awake on guard at night, when the sleep center is in undisputed control of his brain. As guard duty in the military has never gained much popularity, complaints of excessive sleepiness as grounds for exemption are usually viewed with a somewhat jaundiced eye. Over the years we have examined numerous soldiers in our laboratory who had difficulty in meeting the demands of military duty because of excessive sleepiness. In some of them, the wakefulness level was perfectly normal, but there were also those whose complaints were genuine and who suffered from idiopathic excessive sleep.

We do not know why certain people are sleepier than others. As the balance between sleep and wakefulness depends on the activities of two systems of the brain, one overseeing sleep and the other wakefulness, it is entirely possible that a tendency to "sleepiness" depends on the relative effectiveness of the sleep and wakefulness centers in the brain. A further possibility is that the hypocretin level in the brain of the "sleepyheads" is different. We usually do not offer treatment to people who are afflicted with idiopathic excessive sleep, but recommend that they observe proper sleep hygiene. We also explain their limitations regarding the ability to maintain a normal level of wakefulness in situations of sleeplessness.

Chronic Tiredness

Even if we consider all the syndromes and illnesses described so far, there is nothing in them that can explain the large number of people who complain of chronic fatigue. Why is it that so many people complain of constant tiredness? The answer is disappointing in its simplicity: they just don't sleep enough! Modern humans living in an industrialized society sleep far less than their great-grandfathers did a hundred years ago. The invention of the electric light bulb liberated human beings from the burden of the night. With the flick of a switch the working day invades the domain of sleep and pushes it back into the early hours of the morning, and even into daytime. There are so many activities that do not stop during the night: factories, transport and health services, and communications systems go on working unceasingly. Sleep is not taken into account when planning the operation of vast systems that work as a *perpetuum mobile*. Continuous, uninterrupted activity has become a trademark that is worn with pride—Tel Aviv, for example, glories in being Israel's "city without a break," and New York is known the world over as "the city that never sleeps."

Chronic tiredness is what happens when the population of the industrialized world has a vast number of sleep hours owed to it. Every one of us sleeps about an hour or two less than we need to maintain an optimal level of wakefulness during the day. In the Sleep in America national survey of adults conducted by the U.S. National Sleep Foundation in 2001, almost one-third of the respondents (31 percent) said that they get less than 7 hours of sleep per night during the week. The average hours of sleep during weekdays was 7.0, and it increased to 7.8 hours on the weekend. The survey showed that the number of hours of sleep each night is a predictor of daytime sleepiness. The fewer hours slept, the higher percentage of respondents reported sleepiness at a level that interferes with their daily activities. Of people who slept for 7 or 8 hours, roughly 35 percent reported experiencing this kind of tiredness at least a few times per month, but in those who slept only 6 hours, more than 45 percent did, and in those who slept less than 6 hours the figure was over 55 percent.

Tom Wehr, a sleep researcher from the National Institutes of Health in the United States, reversed the relationship between the hours of daylight and darkness in normal youngsters who slept for 6 or 7 hours a night. In the course of several months, instead of being in darkness for 8 hours and in the light for 16, they were asked to go to bed in the dark for 16 hours and were allowed out of bed for 8 hours of daylight. When the amount of time they had slept in the dark was examined, exactly how much the youngsters were enduring a chronic shortage of sleep became clear. In the first days of long nights they slept for more than 9 hours, almost certainly compensating for the long period of chronic deprivation during the daylight hours. They later steadied at 8.5 hours of sleep a night, a sleep quota that apparently reflected their biological need.

Two recently published books have been devoted to modern humans' inconsiderate attitude toward their sleep needs. In *Sleep Thieves,* Stanley Coren enumerates the unavoidable consequences of a shortfall in sleep hours on people's daily wakefulness levels, road and work accidents, work efficiency, and quality of life in general. Like Coren, Bill Dement, the high priest of sleep research in the United States, springs to the defense of sleep's lost respect in his book *The Promise of Sleep,* calling upon all of us to return to the sleep habits of our forebears. Dement's book is possibly the most detailed and enthusiastic defense ever written on the importance of sleep.

It is clear that many people suffer from excessive sleepiness and chronic fatigue because they sleep less than their biological needs demand. This fact should be borne in mind when anyone complains about his or her daily wakefulness level. To anybody complaining of daytime sleepiness and chronic fatigue, the first question should be, "How many hours do you sleep at night?"

12

Children and Sleep Apnea

It is customary to say of someone sleeping peacefully that they are sleeping like a child, or sleeping like a baby. Throughout history, artists have often used the image of a sleeping child or baby to express tranquillity and serenity. But children with sleep breathing disorders are not enjoying tranquil rest.

In the late 1970s, when we struggled to heighten the Israeli medical community's awareness of the existence of sleep disordered breathing, I used to incorporate a short film into my lectures. The film documented the sleep of a six-year-old boy before he underwent a tonsillectomy and after it. The film was shot at the child's home with an old eight-millimeter camera, and it was very dramatic. Before the operation, the child suffered apneas as soon as he fell asleep, and they would sometimes last as long as a minute. To viewers of the film, the apneas seemed to last an eternity, especially as the child could be seen fighting for each breath with every muscle in his body. At the end of every apnea, he would resume his breathing with several deep and loud breaths that produced sighs of relief from the viewers, many of whom feared that the child was going to die of suffocation in his sleep. We returned to his home a few days after he had undergone an operation to remove the tonsils that had been blocking his pharynx. We found a changed child, or as his mother described it, "We have a new child." The child's sleep was peaceful, his

snoring had disappeared, and his breathing was regular and uninterrupted. His behavior during the day had also improved beyond recognition. The child's sleepiness had vanished, and his kindergarten teacher
reported that his ability to concentrate had improved significantly. With
hindsight, the film had a great impact on the attitudes of many doctors
toward sleep apnea syndrome. Even the skeptics among them, who had
viewed breathing disorders during sleep as a medical anecdote associated only with snoring, changed their stance after viewing the film.

Convincing the medical community of the importance of sleep
apnea syndrome in children was difficult not only in Israel. Among the
first people to be diagnosed with sleep apnea syndrome at Stanford University's sleep laboratory were a thirteen-year-old girl and an eleven-
year-old boy. Both suffered from excessive daytime sleepiness despite
sufficient hours of sleep during the night, as well as from hypertension,
which in the boy's case became so severe that there was a real fear for his
life. Examination of both children at the sleep laboratory showed severe
sleep apnea syndrome that required immediate treatment. However,
Guilleminault and Dement were unable to convince their pediatrician
colleagues that the hypertension was caused by sleep apneas that required urgent treatment. It was only after signs of kidney and heart disease were discovered in the boy that they were allowed to treat the children. Both children underwent tracheostomies in 1972, which led to the
complete disappearance of daytime sleepiness and, even more impressive,
to lower blood pressure within twenty-four hours after the operation!

Sleep apnea syndrome in children is different from the syndrome
in adults. The reasons for the condition, as well as its characteristics, effects, and forms of treatment vary significantly. First, unlike adults, where
the syndrome is much more prevalent in men than in women, in children
there is no distinction in prevalence between boys and girls. At the Technion's sleep laboratories more than two thousand children have been diagnosed with sleep disordered breathing, half of them boys and half
girls. Second, despite individual cases that might be described as "Pickwickian children," namely children with a combination of obesity and
excessive sleepiness, obesity in children is not a significant risk factor for
sleep breathing disorders. Children suffer to a lesser degree than adults
from obstructive apneas, and more from partial obstructions that fre-

quently appear during REM sleep. In fact, almost half the apneas in children occur during REM sleep, which occupies only a quarter of total sleep time.

Another distinction is in the effect of apneas on the course of sleep. Whereas in adults these apneas cause repeated interruption in sleep continuity and subsequently to a significant decrease in deep sleep and REM sleep, children do not usually wake up after apneas, so the structure of their sleep is less affected. This is probably the reason why children with sleep disordered breathing are affected less than adults by excessive sleepiness. Furthermore, parents of children with sleep breathing disorders frequently complain that their children have been blessed with excess energy. They present over-alertness, restlessness, fidgeting, and attention difficulties. This depiction corresponds with a diagnosis of attention disorders and hyperactivity, or attention deficit hyperactivity disorder (ADHD), conditions that are usually treated pharmacologically. To date, however, the majority of accounts about the connection between hyperactivity and apneas during sleep in children have been merely anecdotal, and not based on controlled studies. Further research is required to prove a causal connection, and to examine whether treatment of apneas during sleep improves the attention abilities of children with ADHD.

A significant risk factor for breathing disorders during sleep in children is obstruction of the upper airways, which can be caused by enlarged tonsils, adenoids, or obstructions in the nasal cavities—all of which are highly prevalent in children with sleep apnea. The tonsils are two masses of lymphoid tissue in the throat's mucous membrane, located between the palate arches and the tongue, standing like sentries at the gateway to the pharynx. The adenoids are located at the base of the nose.

Sleep disorders in children who have a "blocked nose" and enlarged tonsils did not elude otolaryngologists (ear, nose, and throat specialists) at the beginning of the twentieth century. Sleep disorders in snoring children were meticulously documented, along with their effect on daily functions. In a lecture to the British Medical Association in 1889 titled "On Some Causes of Backwardness and Stupidity in Children," William Hill stated that "the stupid-looking, lazy child who frequently suffers from headaches at school, breathes through his mouth

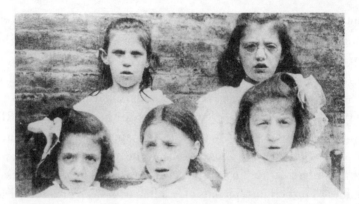

Girls with adenoids, from Walter Moore's *People's Health*
(New York, McMillan, 1913)

instead of his nose, snores and is restless at night, and wakes up with a
dry mouth in the morning, is well worthy of the solicitous attention of
the school medical officer." At the same conference, an otolaryngologist
from Amsterdam named Guye presented a similar paper claiming that
"were it known how many of the children who suffer from chronic
headaches and inability to learn or perform any mental task, also suffer
from chronic nose diseases, a large proportion of these cases could readily be cured." These observations were not reserved only to individual
doctors. In his comprehensive treatise on diseases of the nose and throat
in 1896, Francke H. Bosworth described with great accuracy the suspensions of breathing in children with enlarged tonsils who also had frequent nightmares. The call by Hill, Guye, and Bosworth to examine
every child who is slow to develop and backward in school, to discover
whether they snore or have difficulties breathing during sleep, was reit-
erated about a hundred years later by a young doctor in New Orleans.

Kayshan's Tonsils

David Gozal studied medicine at the Hebrew University in Jerusalem.
After completing his specialization in pediatrics at Bnei Zion Medical
Center in Haifa, he went to the United States. He spent a few years re-

searching cot death together with Ron Harper in Los Angeles, and then joined Tulane University in New Orleans, where he established a laboratory to study the sleep of infants and children. Gozal's interest in the connection between sleep disordered breathing and academic performance was aroused by chance, following treatment of an eight-year-old boy named Kayshan who had severe asthma. Kayshan lived with his mother and four sisters in one of the poorer neighborhoods of New Orleans. Since his mother was not diligent in administering his medication on time, his condition occasionally worsened. He was admitted to the hospital's intensive care unit fourteen times in 1985 due to severe asthma attacks. His hospital discharge chart stated that Kayshan was not receiving proper care for his asthma, was a poor student, was in first grade in spite of his third-grade age, appeared to suffer from attention disorders and hyperactivity, and was frequently disruptive at school. His teachers raised the possibility that Kayshan might be mentally retarded, but his mother would not consent to an examination to diagnose it. No one asked Kayshan's mother, or Kayshan himself, how he slept at night.

The first time Gozal visited Kayshan's room at the hospital, he found him asleep on the floor with his head propped against the bed, snoring heavily and experiencing frequent apneas. It was apparent to Gozal that Kayshan suffered from sleep apnea syndrome. His sisters confirmed that he slept in this manner every night at home too. Since his mother and one of his sisters snored loudly, no one regarded Kayshan's snoring as unusual. Sleep recordings showed that Kayshan had a severe breathing disorder: the boy had almost forty apneas per hour. The day after the sleep examination, Kayshan underwent a tonsillectomy. Three months later he and his mother came for a checkup at Dr. Gozal's clinic. The dramatic change in the boy was plainly evident. His mother related that his illness had improved significantly, even though he was still not taking his medication on time. She proudly showed Gozal her son's latest report card. Kayshan had been moved to second grade and his teachers had written: "It's a miracle. Kayshan is doing well at school and has stopped being disruptive!"

Gozal does not believe in miracles. He was convinced that the remarkable improvement in Kayshan's studies and behavior was a direct result of the improvement in his sleep following the removal of his tonsils. The success of this treatment convinced Gozal that there were more children in the poorer neighborhoods of New Orleans who suffered from breathing disorders during sleep, resulting in poor scholastic performance, and he decided to locate them. He used a laptop computer to construct a monitor for measuring respiration and blood oxygen levels during sleep, enlisted the assistance of his son's classmates, instructed them on use of the instrument, and set out. Gozal visited ninety-seven public schools throughout New Orleans and asked the first-grade teachers in each school to identify their weakest students for him, but many were initially reluctant to help him as his request seemed a little strange. To elicit their consent and cooperation he volunteered to give a lesson on health education in every class whose teacher agreed to cooperate with him. Once the weak students were identified, Gozal contacted their parents and asked to visit them at home so he could record their respiratory functions during sleep. Many parents agreed, especially when they discovered that the examination was free. Equipped with a team of dedicated research assistants from his son Ya'ir's high school, Gozal paid nocturnal visits to the homes of 297 children.

The recordings were successful overall, with the exception of one or two hitches, like the time one of the children's dogs chewed through the electrode wires, or when one sleepwalking child dragged the recording instruments with him through the whole house. Analysis of the nocturnal recordings showed fifty-four children who suffered from sleep apnea, in addition to sixty-six who snored loudly. All were offered tonsillectomies, but only twenty-four of the children afflicted with sleep apnea actually underwent the operation. In the remaining cases, the parents refused the treatment. A year later, the academic performance of the children who had the operation was reviewed, and the findings justified the extensive effort invested in the study. The performance of the children who had undergone surgery had improved significantly compared with their performance in first grade, whereas no improvement was evident in the children whose parents had refused treatment.

The dramatic findings on the connection between breathing disorders during sleep and scholastic achievement made Gozal wonder whether breathing disorders that occur during critical periods in children's intellectual development can affect performance at a later age, too, when their tonsils have diminished in size and respiratory functions during sleep have improved.

Gozal searched for an answer in Jefferson County, Kentucky, after he moved to the University of Louisville. He and his research partner, Dennis Pope, examined the computerized databases of the county's schools and found one thousand adolescents aged thirteen and fourteen whose scholastic performance was significantly poorer than that of their peers. The researchers then selected for each of them a child of similar sex, age, ethnic background, school attended, and street of residence, but whose school grades were high. A detailed questionnaire was sent to the parents of each of the two thousand adolescents asking whether the children had snored in their sleep between ages two and six, whether they had undergone a tonsillectomy at the time due to snoring, and whether they snored now. The parents were unaware of the study's purpose or the researchers' hypotheses. The questionnaires were completed by 83 percent of the parents, and analysis showed that 13 percent of the poor-performance adolescents had snored loudly "almost daily" during infancy, compared with 5 percent of the high-performance adolescents. Twenty-four percent of the under-performers had undergone a tonsillectomy in infancy "due to snoring," compared with only 7 percent of the high-performers.

Assuming that nightly loud snoring is a clear indication of sleep disordered breathing, the extraordinary significance of these findings is that breathing disorders during infancy are liable to cause irreversible damage to the central nervous system, and consequently to lead to learning difficulties at a later age. Further research is undoubtedly required to confirm this hypothesis and to examine whether damage at a later age can be prevented with proper treatment during infancy.

Down Syndrome and Breathing

Down syndrome, which is caused by a congenital genetic defect, is also a risk for breathing disorders in children. This is because Down syndrome is characterized by craniofacial anomalies that narrow the airways, particularly a small lower jaw and a large and thickened tongue. Children with Down syndrome are also prone to frequent infections of the airways resulting in inflammation of the tonsils, which exacerbates the narrowing of the upper airways around the pharynx. Several studies have revealed a high prevalence of sleep breathing disorders in Down syndrome children, one of which was conducted at our laboratory by Dana Pillar. Pillar interviewed the parents of 120 Down syndrome children and examined 18 of them at the sleep laboratory. According to the interviews, one in every four children snored loudly during the night and had a clear tendency toward sleepiness during the day. The sleep laboratory examinations showed more than ten apneas per hour of sleep in 90 percent of the children who complained of snoring and sleepiness. Children who underwent surgery at an early age to remove tonsils or shorten the tongue complained less of snoring and sleepiness, and their sleep was normal.

In the 1930s and 1940s it was customary to operate on every case of tonsillitis, including the mildest ones, which made tonsillectomy the most common of operations. In the 1960s, medical wisdom shifted, discounting the operation except in extreme cases, claiming that tonsils would shrink of their own accord with age. The success of tonsillectomies and adenoidectomies in treating sleep breathing disorders in children has changed medical attitudes toward these operations. Nowadays, sleep examinations are critical in diagnosing sleep apnea and other breathing disorders, and tonsillectomy is accepted as an effective treatment for these problems, especially in Down syndrome patients.

Crib Death

Adult patients with sleep apnea syndrome rarely die of suffocation in their sleep. Even when apneas last for ninety seconds and longer, the brain's emergency systems ensure that the patient wakes up in time and resumes breathing. Infants, however, do sometimes die in their sleep. In one out of every thousand families, an infant dies in its sleep, in most cases during its second to fourth months of life.

The death of infants during sleep has been known for thousands of years. The story of a woman who has lost her baby during sleep is related in the Judgment of Solomon: "And this woman's child died in the night; because she overlay it" (I Kings 3:19). This concise phrase enfolds within it the tragedy of accidental killing of infants, which was apparently quite common to the ancients. At a time when parents and children slept in the same bed, it was not unusual for one of the parents to roll over in their sleep and unwittingly cover the infant with their body and smother it to death. In the eighteenth century, infant death in this manner was termed *Opressio infantis*.

It became apparent only during the nineteenth century that accidental suffocation by parents could not explain every infant death during sleep. The phenomenon was not formally described until 1969, when it was given the name sudden infant death syndrome, informally known as crib death, and defined as "the sudden death of an infant or young child, which is unexpected by (medical) history, and in which a thorough postmortem examination fails to demonstrate an adequate cause of death." The definition was later restricted to deaths of infants up to the age of one year.

The prevalence of crib death varies from country to country, and even within countries and between different ethnic and social groups. In Israel, the incidence is approximately 0.4 to 0.8 cases in every 1,000 births; in the United States, 1.4 cases in 1,000 births; and in France, about 2 cases in every 1,000 births. In some countries this figure runs as high as 6 in every 1,000. Incidence is higher in premature infants, infants born to mothers who used drugs during pregnancy, and infants born to mothers from the lower socioeconomic classes. Eighty-five percent of deaths occur during the first six months of life; 61 percent occur between the third and sixth months of the infant's life. Data from various sources throughout the world show that the number of boys who die of the syndrome is higher than the number of girls, and the majority of cases occur in the winter months.

What is the cause of crib death? There is much evidence showing that a large number of deaths are caused by apneas during sleep. Unlike adults, who escape suspensions of breathing by waking up, infants do not wake up and may die of suffocation.

The first paper to assert that the cause of crib death is suspension of breathing during sleep turned out to be a terrible mistake. In October 1972, the pediatrician Alfred Steinschneider published a paper in an American pediatrics journal describing the crib deaths of two infants, Molly and Noah Hoyt, from New York. Three of their siblings had died earlier, apparently under similar circumstances. Steinschneider reported that prior to their deaths the two children had suffered protracted apneas during sleep, which were discovered by physiological recordings made during their hospitalization, and they died a short time after being discharged. Steinschneider's paper, indicating apneas as the cause of death and the possibility of a familial propensity toward crib death, has been widely quoted by researchers. But a skeptical district attorney who happened upon the paper in 1986 reached a very different conclusion. He suspected that the evidence pointed to murder rather than crib death. Following an extensive investigation, the children's mother confessed to murdering her five children and was brought to trial in 1994. Although she retracted her confession during the trial, the jury found her guilty. Steinschneider testified on her behalf at the trial.

The Hoyt case somewhat undermined the belief that crib death is caused by apneas, although there is further evidence to support the hypothesis regarding the connection. The most solid evidence is in infants who have survived suffocating in their sleep at the last moment. In these cases, parents would find their baby lying in its bed, face blue from lack of oxygen, wheezing, and trying with all its might to resume breathing. If the parents arrived just a little later, the baby would be found as white as chalk, its body slack, unconscious, and its heartbeat very slow. Only vigorous resuscitation efforts can bring these babies back to life. Observations of infants who have survived show that they are at greater risk of crib death than those who do not have such a history—almost one in every ten infants who died in their sleep had experienced a case of "near death" before the fatal incident. Based on these observations, researchers believe that two-thirds of crib death victims died as a result of a prolonged apnea during sleep.

Various findings indicate that there is no single cause of apneas during sleep in infants, but a combination of factors. Some of these have to do with physiological changes that occur during the first six months of life, both in sleep and in the mechanisms controlling the cardiorespiratory system, and other factors are connected to possible defects in a number of mechanisms that prevent the infant from efficiently combating life-threatening episodes during sleep. At least some of these malfunctions connect crib death and sleep apnea syndrome, in both children and adults.

In contrast to the sleep of adults, which is composed of several defined stages distinct from each other in the brain's electrical activity and the activity of the autonomic nervous system, an infant's sleep during the first months of life is not organized. There are two kinds of sleep in infants: quiet sleep, characterized by regular breathing, regular heartbeat, and absence of body movement, and active sleep, in which respiratory instability, frequent variations in heart rate, rapid eye movement, and numerous muscular spasms can be observed. As infants grow older, quiet sleep comprises stages 1, 2, 3, and 4, defined as non-REM sleep, whereas active sleep becomes REM sleep or dream sleep. The appearance of very brief apneas, up to ten seconds long during active sleep, is a physiological occurrence that gradually disappears as the infant develops. Occasionally, brief apneas can be detected during dream sleep in adults too.

Sleep That Is Too Deep

Several studies have examined whether the sleep of infants who have died in their cribs differed from the sleep of healthy ones. Statistics predict one death in every thousand births; hence, if physiological records were to be kept on ten thousand infants during the first month of life, about ten would be expected to fall victim to crib death. Examination of sleep records made on these infants could perhaps reveal the possible reasons.

One of the most notable studies on the sleep of crib death infants was conducted in Britain for one year beginning in July 1980. Respiration and heartbeat records were maintained for 6,914 infants, 2,337 of whom were premature, during the first month of life. Twenty-nine of the infants fell victim to crib death. None of the physiological records of these infants, however, showed any prolonged apneas during sleep, and except for one infant no disorders of any kind were found in the heart's electrical activity.

Ron Harper's research group from the University of California at Los Angeles also studied crib death, first looking at how the sleep of infants at high risk of crib death differed from that of infants who were not at risk. Children considered at high risk for crib death included premature babies, infants who had survived suffocation during sleep, and siblings of infants who had died of the syndrome.

Harper and his colleagues conducted sleep recordings on twenty-five healthy infants and twenty-five siblings of infants who had died, tracking the sleep structure, heartbeat, and respiration rate of both groups for the first week of life, and every month thereafter up to the age of six months. They discovered, as had their British colleagues, that there are no dramatic differences in the sleep data for the two groups. Yet, equipped with expertise he had acquired in studying the development of heart and respiration rhythms during the first six months of life, Harper approached David Southall, the head of the British research group, and asked him to forward his team's records for further analysis in Los Angeles. A doctoral student, Vicki Schechtman, handled the data processing, which shed new light on the British study's findings.

Schechtman, Harper, and their colleagues found that although crib death victims did not show any obvious signs of distress in the first weeks of life, there were a number of unusual features in their respiration and heartbeat records. These findings suggested that the respiratory and cardiovascular response system had been more rigid in the infants who fell victim to crib death than in the ones that developed normally. This was manifested in their respiratory rhythm not changing in response to a rise or fall in blood pressure, whereas the respiratory rhythm in normal infants increased or decreased. Moreover, the heartbeat was insufficiently flexible to respond to changes in respiration or wakefulness levels in the infants who had died. Their sleep had also been deeper, which could be surmised from the fact that they experienced fewer of the brief awakenings that characterize the sleep of infants, especially during the transitions from "quiet" to "active" sleep. Paradoxically, fewer brief apneas had been recorded in the infants who died than in those who didn't.

This combination of findings led Harper and his colleagues to the conclusion that crib death victims were unable to efficiently respond to dangerous apneas, including waking up in time to resume breathing. This conclusion confirmed accounts from parents of infants who had survived suffocation during sleep, who reported that their children's sleep was very deep, and it was difficult to wake them up. (After finishing her doctorate, Schechtman continued to do useful research on crib death until 1998, when she died, at only forty-two, of complications during treatment of leukemia.)

Similar findings regarding deep sleep were also reported in infants who were at risk of crib death. In siblings of crib death victims, for example, whose risk is four times higher than that of other children, fewer awakenings were recorded from two to three months of age than in a control group.

One hypothesis is that crib death and sleep apnea syndrome may have certain hereditary factors in common. Although no controlled studies on the connection have been conducted, there are several anecdotal cases on record. In 1978, Kingman Strohl and his colleagues published a report in the *New England Journal of Medicine* on five brothers, two of whom snored in their sleep and suffered from excessive sleepiness, one who was a known chronic snorer and died in his sleep at age thirty, one who was also a known chronic snorer, and one who was healthy and had no disorders of any kind. The father, who had abandoned his family long before the study, snored very loudly and was sleepy for most hours of the day, according to the mother. One of the brother's daughters died in her crib at the age of four months.

There is also evidence that infants who experienced non-fatal apneas during the first months of life endured sleep apnea syndrome as adults. Christian Guilleminault and his group from Stanford observed twenty-five infants aged between a few months and five years, who were selected from a group of seven hundred infants that had survived suffocation during sleep. At five years of age, all the infants suffered from sleep apnea syndrome, and there was a high incidence of the syndrome in their families.

The possible connection between sleep apnea and crib death necessitates special attention to infants born to families with a history of sleep apnea, especially when more than one family member is afflicted with the syndrome.

Back to Sleeping on the Back

The absence of warning signs for high risk of crib death makes it difficult to contend with the syndrome. The death of an infant usually descends on parents out of the blue and arouses feelings of helplessness and despair. One of the methods of dealing with the risk of crib death is using sleep monitoring instruments that set off an alarm if an extreme change occurs in a sleeping infant's breathing or heartbeat. Despite the wide use of monitors, very few studies have examined their efficacy, and the most comprehensive study on the subject has only recently been published.

In 2001, Rangasamy Ramanathan and his colleagues reported on an extensive study of the use of home monitors in more than a thousand infants, including healthy babies, premature babies, infants who had survived suffocation, and siblings of crib death infants. Based on over 700,000 hours of recordings, the researchers concluded that apneas during sleep are reasonably common in infants, regardless of risk factors. Twenty percent of the healthy infants had apneas at a prevalence similar to that of infants in the risk group. In contrast, occurrences that were defined as extreme, namely prolonged apneas, were recorded only in premature babies up to the age of forty-three weeks from start of gestation. The researchers concluded that based on these findings it was impossible to determine the efficacy of nocturnal monitoring, or to determine which of the infants required monitoring.

Studies in some countries have tried to analyze the cause of death in a large number of crib fatalities, and they have revealed a limited number of environmental risk factors. The most important appears to be the infant's position during sleep. Second, having a mother who smoked doubled the risk of crib death; third, overheating of the bedroom was also associated with increased risk. Susan Beal, from Adelaide, Australia, first made the observation that infant victims of crib death were most commonly found lying on their abdomens. Subsequent studies showed that infants who slept on their stomach had three to nine times higher risk of crib death than infants who slept on their side or back.

Based on these findings, several countries launched campaigns in the 1990s to persuade parents to put their infants to sleep on their backs. Beal herself led the first "back to sleep" campaign in Tasmania, Australia, and many followed in her footsteps. In some countries, the campaigns have been a resounding success. In the United States, at the start of the effort in 1992, 73 percent of children slept on their stomachs; two years later the number had been reduced to 43 percent. Similar changes have been recorded in Australia, New Zealand, Scandinavia, England, and several other European countries. In most of these countries the number of crib deaths dropped. In New Zealand, for example, the number declined from 4.4 to 2.1 deaths in every 1,000 children. In England, too, there was a decrease of over 50 percent. Although there is still no explanation for why sleeping on the stomach might be more dangerous than on the back, the assumption is that it is connected to blockage of the airways by pillows or mattresses. Most infants will wake up if they experience respiratory distress, but infants who have a malfunction in the respiratory mechanism or the awakening mechanisms are liable to not wake up.

13

Sleep Apnea, the Heart, and the Blood Vessels

The first researchers to make sleep records of Pickwickian patients were aware of the significant effect apneas had on the heart's activity during sleep. Both Gerardy and his colleagues and Gumnit and Drachman reported that the heart rate of Pickwickian patients changed drastically, becoming slower during the apneas and greatly accelerating with the resumption of breathing. Later, Lugaresi and his colleagues showed similar changes in general and pulmonary blood pressure, both of which dropped during apneas and were elevated drastically when breathing resumed. Furthermore, tracheostomy in hypertensive apneic patients sometimes resulted in a dramatic reduction in blood pressure, as was shown in children by the Stanford group.

Nevertheless, it was not known whether apneas during sleep affect the function of the heart and blood vessels during wakefulness. It was clear that Pickwickian patients tend to suffer from cardiovascular disease, but this was ascribed to their excess weight, not to breathing disorders. The Bologna group that found a close association between snoring and high blood pressure in San Marino did not know if the snorers actually suffered from sleep apnea. It was possible that nocturnal apneas are associated with cardiovascular disease, especially in people who are not obese.

One of the first observations on apneas and cardiovascular disease was made at our laboratory, using the data we collected at the end of the 1970s on the prevalence of complaints about daytime sleepiness and chronic fatigue in industrial workers. Our analysis showed that there appeared to be a link between sleep apnea and the prevalence of hypertension. In the workers whose sleep featured more than ten apneas per hour, 36.3 percent had high blood pressure; in those whose sleep was free of apneas, only 7.4 percent were hypertensive. Our report, published in *Sleep,* the official journal of the American Sleep Research Society, in 1983, cautiously suggested that doctors consider the possibility that patients with primary hypertension might also be suffering from sleep apnea syndrome. This association with high blood pressure entirely changed the medical approach to sleep apnea syndrome.

Hypertension has been dubbed "the silent killer" for good reason. Many people live with hypertension for several years without knowing it. In the first stages of the disease, it has no warning signs to alert the patient. In many cases it is discovered only after damage has been done to vital systems, such as the kidneys, blood vessels, heart, and retina.

A distinction is generally made between two main types of hypertension: primary and secondary. Secondary hypertension is caused by a disease, such as kidney disease, hyperactivity of the thyroid gland, or tumors on the adrenal gland. As soon as the primary cause is diagnosed and appropriately treated, blood pressure returns to its normal level. But the cause of the disease can be identified in only 10 to 15 percent of cases. In all remaining cases, no obvious cause can be found for the disease, and this condition is defined as primary hypertension.

Primary hypertension is a result of other factors, such as genetics (because the risk of hypertension is especially high in children of parents with hypertension), age (since the disease appears mostly in people over thirty), or gender (as men are at greater risk for hypertension than women). Race may be a factor, too: studies in the United States have shown that hypertension is more prevalent in African-Americans than in Caucasians. These factors are beyond our control, but others are not, including lifestyle, obesity, alcohol consumption, and salt intake. If we summarize everything we know about these factors, we could say that a very high risk of hypertension will be found in obese people who are physically inactive, are exposed to mental stress, have a fondness for a drop of the hard stuff, and like heavily salted food. Each of these factors constitutes a risk of hypertension, and a combination of them all increases it even more.

Discussion of these factors can be found in almost all medical, scientific, or popular literature on hypertension, but none of these sources ever mention sleep apnea syndrome. To us, however, it seemed significant that the presence of hypertension is five times higher in people with sleep disordered breathing, so we decided to study the subject further. This time we researched the association from the opposite direction: we investigated whether people with hypertension are more prone to breathing disorders during sleep than the general population. For this purpose we recruited fifty hypertension patients so we could make sleep recordings of them. We made no classifications in their selection, simply approaching all the patients who came to the Rambam Medical Center Hypertension Clinic in Haifa on particular days and asking them to spend a night at the sleep laboratory. To our delight, no one refused—all agreed to contribute one of their nights for our research.

The examination findings confirmed our suspicion: in 22 percent of the hypertension patients we found more than ten apneas per hour, a prevalence five times higher than in the general population. Furthermore, these patients had the typical complaints of sleep apnea syndrome, including chronic fatigue, sleepiness, and nightly loud snoring. Since we found no significant variances in age or weight between hypertension patients who have apneas and those who do not, we assumed that there was an association between the apneas and hypertension. Publication of our findings in the *American Heart Journal* in 1984 preceded similar reports from several other laboratories by a number of months. They all pointed to an association between sleep apnea and hypertension.

Although these findings were published in scientific journals of the highest order, it can scarcely be said that they caused much excitement in the medical community outside the small fraternity of sleep researchers. Criticism, in fact, was quick to appear. The primary argument was that obesity is a common risk factor for both hypertension and sleep apnea; therefore, critics claimed, it was almost impossible in hypertension cases to distinguish between the contribution of obesity and that of apneas during sleep. John Wright, an epidemiologist from Yorkshire, England, and his colleagues reviewed fifty-four studies dealing with the association between sleep apnea and hypertension and other heart diseases, and they concluded that no solid evidence exists for the independent influence of sleep apnea on hypertension. Their report, published in the prestigious *British Medical Journal* in 1997, was sharply critical of claims regarding a causal association between apneas and hypertension. Our own statistics, gathered from ten thousand people who were examined at the Technion Sleep Laboratory, clearly demonstrated a direct correlation between the number of apneas during sleep and the prevalence of hypertension. But they also showed an equally direct correlation between body mass and prevalence of hypertension, making it difficult to determine whether the apneas were contributing to hypertension or if it was simply obesity contributing to both the apneas and the hypertension.

Conclusive evidence, however, of a direct association between sleep apneas and hypertension was not long in coming. In the same year as Wright's article in the *BMJ*, Eliot Phillipson of Toronto, whose curiosity had earlier led him to examine the respiratory function of a dog that fell asleep in his laboratory, used his original thinking to devise another experiment that turned out to be critical. Phillipson and his group developed a novel method of simulating sleep apnea syndrome in dogs. They implanted a valve in the dog's throat that alternately opened and closed by means of a radio-transmitted computer command. Closing the valve caused suspensions of breathing in the dog similar to those in sleep apnea patients, and opening it caused removal of the blockage and resumption of breathing. In order to limit the apneas to sleep only, electrodes implanted in the dog's scalp were connected to a tiny amplifier and transmitter that relayed brain waves to a computer in an adjacent room. The computer analyzed the dog's brain waves to determine whether it was asleep or awake. As soon as the brain waves indicated that the dog was asleep, the valve in its throat closed and its breathing was suspended until the moment of awakening. The awakening was received by the computer, which sent a command for the valve to open and allow resumption of breathing.

Phillipson and his colleagues examined the effect of apneas during sleep on the dog's blood pressure during the day and at night. At first, the apneas caused the dog's blood pressure to become elevated by 13 millimeters of mercury, but only during the night. Within a few days, however, there was an elevation of 15 millimeters of mercury in blood pressure during the day too. Since every apnea culminated in an awakening, the team examined the possibility that the frequent awakenings, rather than blockage of the airways, were causing the elevation in blood pressure.

To investigate this, instead of activating the valve and blocking the airways when the dog fell asleep, the researchers awakened the dog by making a loud noise. These awakenings caused an elevation in blood pressure during sleep only, and did not cause any elevation in blood pressure during the day. The findings of Phillipson and his colleagues did not provide an explanation for the fact that apneas during sleep caused an elevation in blood pressure; they only provided direct proof of a causal association between apneas during sleep and hypertension. Within a short time, solid proof of this association was received from studies on people too.

The year 2000 was remarkable for the proliferation of research data on the association between hypertension and sleep apnea syndrome. Between February and August, new scientific papers were published almost every month indicating that sleep apnea syndrome is a risk factor for hypertension. All the papers were published in medical journals of the highest order, and all were based on data gathered from particularly large populations. The first of these papers, published in the *British Medical Journal,* was a joint product of the sleep laboratories at the Technion and in Toronto.

The database at the Technion's Sleep Medicine Center is one of the largest worldwide, but it was impossible to rely on it alone to research the association between hypertension and sleep apnea. Diagnosis of hypertension in patients examined at the Technion's laboratories is based on reports by patients, which are not always reliable, especially when they report that they do not suffer from hypertension. Victor Hoff-stein, head of the laboratory for diagnosis of sleep disorders at Saint Michael's Hospital in Toronto, maintains meticulous blood pressure records for all the patients examined in his laboratory. He measures blood pressure before nocturnal examinations, and again in the morning after patients awaken. At one of the scientific conferences on sleep, he described his system of measuring blood pressure, after which I asked whether he would be willing to collaborate with us on a thorough study of the association between hypertension and sleep apnea. Hoffstein did not hesitate for a second, and with a generosity rare in the scientific world he immediately sent us data on three thousand people who had been ex-amined at his laboratory.

The data turned out to be a treasure trove. First, we discovered how erroneous conclusions about the prevalence of hypertension in sleep apnea patients can be when based only on patient reports. The inaccu-racy was particularly conspicuous in people with severe sleep apnea syn-drome. Only 30 percent of them had reported hypertension, but blood pressure measurements revealed a further 30 percent with blood pres-sure higher than 140/90 millimeters of mercury, values that are consid-ered the upper limit for normal blood pressure. In other words, the per-centage of severe sleep apnea syndrome patients who suffered from hypertension was in fact double the percentage of those who reported it.

Analysis of the data from Toronto and the Technion showed that sleep apnea syndrome is a significant risk factor for hypertension, unre-lated to body weight or other risk factors, such as age, gender, smoking, or alcohol consumption. We could determine that the risk for hyperten-sion in people who have more than thirty apneas during sleep was 50 percent higher than in people of the same demographic characteristics and background illnesses but with fewer than ten episodes per hour. In people whose sleep includes at least sixty episodes per hour, the risk rose to 100 percent and higher. The association between hypertension and the severity of the syndrome in sleep was particularly conspicuous in people aged thirty to sixty, and less conspicuous in younger or older people. (I will elaborate on the possible reasons for this later.)

Because we had accurate data on the medical history of each and every patient, including medical treatment, we were also able to assess the effect of the syndrome's severity on the efficacy of treatment for hypertension. We found about eighty patients whose disease had been ineffectively treated. In other words, despite treatment with medication to reduce blood pressure, frequently with more than one type of medication, measurements of these patients' blood pressure showed higher than normal values. This aspect of hypertension, being resistant to medication, is known in medical literature. For unknown reasons, some people do not respond to medication and continue to have high blood pressure, which can cause irreparable damage. When we compared the group of non-responders with those who benefited from treatment, we found that the only variance between them was the severity of breathing disorders during sleep. Those who did not respond to treatment also had more severe sleep apnea syndrome than the others, with an average of forty-four apneas per hour in the non-responders, compared with thirty-two episodes per hour in those who had been effectively treated.

These findings, as well as additional evidence of the association between treatment-resistant hypertension and sleep apnea syndrome, point to the possibility that sleep breathing disorders cause the lack of response to medication for treatment of hypertension. There is further support for this conclusion in a factor that we shall explore in more detail later: treatment of sleep apnea by introducing forced airflow via the nostrils, it turns out, also reduces blood pressure.

Dippers That Do Not Dip

Analysis of the findings on the Toronto patients revealed additional blood pressure characteristics in sleep apnea patients that can help identify people at high risk for the syndrome.

It has been known for several years that there are significant distinctions between daytime and nighttime blood pressure values. Several studies in which blood pressure was measured with automatic instruments every thirty or sixty minutes over a twenty-four-hour period found that pressures during the day were 10–15 millimeters of mercury higher than at night. These variances were found both in healthy people and in some hypertensive patients, but in other hypertensive patients blood pressure does not vary between daytime and nighttime. People whose blood pressure drops during sleep are called "dippers," and people whose blood pressure does not are "non-dippers." Comparison of the two groups showed that non-dippers are at higher risk than dippers are for heart attack and stroke. The first scientific papers to address these differences did not even consider the possibility that non-dippers may suffer from sleep disordered breathing. We found solid evidence of this in the measurements conducted in Toronto.

When we compared morning and evening blood pressure measurements, we found that patients with severe sleep apnea syndrome had higher morning blood pressure than evening blood pressure, and vice versa—patients with a mild case of the syndrome, or patients who did not have breathing disorders during sleep, had higher evening blood pressure values than in the morning. This observation has practical significance, for these measurements can help indicate which people are at high risk for the syndrome. Other researchers who have carried out frequent daytime and nighttime blood pressure measurements have reported similar findings.

One in the remarkable string of papers on sleep apnea published in 2000 appeared in the *Journal of the American Medical Association* in April. This was the first report on a large cross-sectional research effort known as the American Sleep Heart Health Study, in which many researchers throughout the United States were involved. Its purpose was to evaluate the association between cardiovascular diseases and sleep disordered breathing in a large population. More than six thousand people had their sleep assessed, in their homes, by means of portable polysomnographs. The assessment findings were compared for blood pressure data and prevalence of heart disease. Participants in the study were selected by random sample from the general population. The association between breathing disorders and hypertension in this study was similar to the findings we reported on the population of sleep apnea syndrome patients tested at our sleep laboratory. The greater the number of apneas during sleep, the higher was the risk for hypertension, even after the possible contributions of body weight, neck circumference, age, gender, smoking, and alcohol consumption were taken into consideration. The people whose at-home sleep assessments showed that they experienced at least thirty full or partial apneas per hour were at a 40 percent higher risk for hypertension than those who did not experience any apneas at all. This association held for both men and women.

In May 2000, another paper on hypertension and sleep disordered breathing appeared, this one in the *New England Journal of Medicine*, by Terry Young's group. Their study was a reassessment of 709 people from the Wisconsin sample of civil servants, four years after they had first been tested at the sleep laboratory. People who had recorded at least fifteen respiratory episodes per hour in the first assessment, they found, were at three times the risk of developing hypertension than people who did not experience any breathing disorders during sleep. This risk was unrelated to an increase in body weight, alcohol consumption, or smoking. The great significance of this report was that, whereas other studies had discussed the association between hypertension and sleep apnea syndrome retrospectively, based on information about the patients' past, the study by Young and her colleagues was prospective—the results of sleep assessments were used to forecast the development of hypertension four years later.

The following August, Anthony Kales and Edward Bixler's group in Hershey, Pennsylvania, published yet another article on sleep apnea and hypertension. They studied 1,741 men and women, selected from a population of more than 16,000 people according to complaints and typical symptoms of sleep apnea. Kales and Bixler found that apnea during sleep was an independent risk factor for hypertension, especially in people forty to sixty years old.

By this time the sheer quantity of data accumulated on the association between hypertension and sleep disordered breathing was powerful evidence of a link. Skepticism has faded, and today there is widespread recognition that the possibility of sleep apnea syndrome must be taken into consideration in every case of primary hypertension.

Coronary Heart Disease and Strokes

Coronary heart disease, or cardiac atherosclerosis, is the primary cause of death in the Western world, in both women and men. Like hypertension, cardiac atherosclerosis can be "dormant" for several years before the patient experiences chest pains or has a heart attack caused by full or partial blockage of the bloodstream in the coronary arteries. Sadly, in many cases the first heart attack is also the last. Because hypertension is one of the risk factors for cardiac atherosclerosis, it is hardly surprising that many researchers have focused on a possible association between cardiac atherosclerosis and sleep apnea. The first studies, conducted in the 1980s and 1990s, assessed groups of cardiac atherosclerosis patients in sleep laboratories and found a relatively high prevalence of sleep apnea compared with the general population. In general, sleep apnea syndrome was found at twice the prevalence in cardiac atherosclerosis patients as in people in the control groups, for both men and women. As with hypertension, the association between apneas and heart disease was unrelated to other risk factors for atherosclerosis, such as age, gender, weight, smoking, or alcohol consumption.

An association was found between cardiac atherosclerosis and sleep apnea when it was researched in the opposite direction, too—when the prevalence of heart disease was examined in a population of sleep apnea syndrome patients. The percentage of people suffering from coronary heart disease among sleep apnea patients is between 10 and 15 percent, and only about 5 percent in the general population. In other words, there are twice to three times the number of heart patients among sleep apnea patients than in the general population.

Some findings indicate that sleep apnea is a risk factor for atherosclerosis in general, not only for cardiac atherosclerosis. A study from Limoges in France showed that patients suffering from general atherosclerosis experienced breathing disorders during sleep at four times the prevalence of people with no sclerotic findings. A study conducted at the University of California in Los Angeles found that 21.3 percent of forty-seven sleep apnea syndrome patients had partial blockage of the carotid artery, which carries blood to the brain, compared with only 2.5 percent among the control patients of the same age. A further cause of stroke, atheroma of the carotid artery's wall, is also more prevalent in sleep apnea syndrome patients.

Epidemiological studies, especially from Scandinavia, found that people who had suffered a stroke caused by blockage of one of the brain's arteries reported regular nightly snoring at a much greater frequency than the control groups. The highest risk for stroke was found in men who snored nightly and were hypertensive. An even higher risk was found in people who had suffered a stroke and reported symptoms of sleep apnea syndrome, such as excessive sleepiness. These epidemiological findings are supported by sleep assessments carried out on people who have had a stroke. The assessments reveal a higher prevalence of sleep apnea in these patients than in healthy people of the same age and body mass. More than ten apneas per hour of sleep were found in almost half the people who had suffered a stroke. Reports by sleep apnea patients about regular snoring long before the stroke indicate that sleep breathing disorders preceded the stroke and were not a result of it.

The American Sleep Heart Health Study also provided evidence of an association between sleep disordered breathing and cardiovascular disease. Its findings were surprising. This study showed that even a relatively small number of apneas during sleep was associated with a significant risk for heart disease.

The main limitation of all the studies described so far is their retrospective nature: in almost all of them, sleep assessments were conducted after the stroke or heart attack, and no information is available on the quality of the patients' sleep before they contracted the disease. Although snoring prior to the event might indicate that breathing disorders preceded the disease, it should be remembered that not all snorers stop breathing during their sleep. To prove a causal association between sleep breathing disorders and cardiovascular disease, a prospective study is required. A study of this kind would follow up large populations of sleep apnea patients and healthy people over several years in order to monitor strokes or heart attacks, as was done in the sample of Wisconsin civil servants and the American Sleep Heart Health Study. Findings from studies of this kind will teach us a great deal about the effect of sleep apnea on the cardiovascular system.

Deadly Dreams

Several studies have shown that the risk for a heart attack is not constant at all hours of the day. A relatively large number of heart attacks occur during sleep, especially in the early hours of the morning toward awakening and during the first few hours after awakening. Is it possible that there is a link between apneas during sleep and a relatively high prevalence of heart attacks at this time of day? A convenient method of following the function of the heart during sleep is by recording its electrical activity with an electrocardiograph, or ECG. Variations in ECG recordings during sleep might indicate a disorder in the activity of the heart due to defective blood supply (ischemia) to the cardiac muscle, or disruption of the activity of the cells that regulate the heart's contractions. Studies assessing ECG readings during sleep in patients with coronary heart disease and sleep apnea found many more pathological changes in them than in people with only heart disease or only sleep apnea. Changes in ECG readings indicating ischemia usually appeared toward the end of the episode, immediately upon resumption of breathing, when heart rate and physical exertion were at their highest. At this time, the heart pump requires large quantities of blood for its operation, more than the coronary arteries are able to supply. This causes distress to the cardiac muscle, as indicated by the pathological symptoms on the electrical recordings of its activity.

Dr. Nir Peled joined the Technion's sleep laboratory staff in his first year of medical studies, and for his doctoral thesis he conducted a study of heart patients who also had sleep apnea syndrome. He found that the patients whose ECG recordings showed nocturnal ischemia episodes had more severe sleep apnea syndrome than the patients in whom no nocturnal ischemia was observed. Moreover, effective treatment of the syndrome significantly reduced the number of ischemic events. Other researchers have shown that cardiac ischemia episodes in sleep apnea patients tended to occur during dream sleep. This phase of sleep is characterized by vigorous activity of the sympathetic nervous system, which increases the demand for blood supply to the cardiac muscle, causing its functional disruption.

These findings, indicating that the combination of heart disease and sleep disordered breathing involves a higher risk for heart attack during sleep than each of these diseases on its own, recently gained direct support. Jan Hedner's group from Gothenburg in Sweden followed up sixty-two coronary heart disease patients, nineteen of whom were also afflicted with sleep apnea syndrome, over a period of five years. At the end of this time, Hedner and his colleagues found that 37.5 percent of the heart patients who also suffered from sleep apnea had died as a result of a heart attack, compared with only 9.3 percent of the patients who were free of sleep apneas. Statistical analysis showed that apneas during sleep were associated with mortality irrespective of the other risk factors, such as age, gender, type of medical treatment, and body weight.

In short, there is much evidence today that sleep apnea syndrome, far beyond its disruptive effects in the form of snoring, disgruntled spouses, continual tiredness, falling asleep in meetings or at the wheel of a moving vehicle, and ruining your sex life, can also exert a much more deadly influence. It can also kill.

14

From Baroreceptors to Free Radicals

The prevalence in sleep apnea patients of hypertension, strokes, coronary cardiac diseases, and calcification of the carotid artery is an indication that the syndrome is a risk factor for cardiovascular diseases in general. What, then, is the risk factor common to all the diseases linked to the heart and blood vessels in sleep apnea syndrome patients? In recent years numerous studies have investigated the physiological mechanisms involved in increased cardiovascular disease in these patients. The two most prominent of these mechanisms, the studies have revealed, are the autonomic nervous system, particularly the subsystem known as the sympathetic autonomic system, and the complicated cellular processes that lead to atherosclerosis.

A Neural Storm

One possible reason why sleep breathing disorders could help cause cardiovascular disease is the intensified activity of the autonomic nervous system, during both sleep and wakefulness. The autonomic nervous system encompasses two subsystems: the sympathetic and the parasympathetic nervous systems, which balance each other.

The sympathetic system goes into action in situations of stress, when there is a call for vigorous and immediate physical action. It is responsible for the distending of the blood vessels taking blood to the skeletal muscles and the contraction of those taking blood to the internal organs, so that blood pressure is increased. It does this by releasing adrenaline into the bloodstream, which heightens respiratory and heart rates, dilates the pupils, and increases muscle tension. The structure of the sympathetic system enables it to simultaneously affect a large number of other systems so that all these changes take place at the same time. The activity of the sympathetic system is overseen by brain centers in the hypothalamus that are interconnected by chains of ganglia, which are masses of nerve cells running the length of the spinal column and along both sides of it.

The parasympathetic nervous system, in contrast, is a "moderating" system, the action of which reduces muscular activity and slows the heart and respiratory rates. The parasympathetic system takes over when a person falls asleep, reducing the heart and respiratory rates and slackening the skeletal muscles. But the picture changes radically with the transition to REM sleep. In the blink of an eye, radical changes take place in the respiratory and heart rates and blood pressure, evidence of vigorous action being taken by the sympathetic system. If we didn't know that a person was asleep at this stage, the physiological recordings would convince us that he or she was in the middle of some vigorous physical activity.

The delicate balance between the two autonomic subsystems, which determines that each of them is in control for only part of sleeping time, is completely upset by sleep apnea syndrome. The activity of the sympathetic system in sleep apnea patients is not restricted to REM sleep, as in normal functioning, but instead intrudes into all the sleep stages. This is because the termination of each apnea is accompanied by the vigorous activation of the sympathetic system, which is rallied each time the brain's control mechanisms identify a drop in the blood oxygen saturation level, which might impair a sufficient supply of oxygen to the body's tissues. A reduction in the oxygen level and a rise in the carbon dioxide level cause the reflexive and vigorous activation of the sympathetic system, and especially of the system's fibers connected to the body's muscles. Their activation causes the swift contraction of the blood vessels, which in turn causes elevated blood pressure. This disruption of the balance between the two autonomic systems explains why, in at least some sleep apnea patients, there is no reduction of blood pressure during sleep, as we have seen.

Two studies have proved that apneas during sleep cause the activation of the sympathetic neural fibers. Jan Hedner, from Sweden, and Virend Somer, who today is at the Mayo Clinic in Rochester, Minnesota, led these two studies, in which their research groups inserted tiny electrodes into the sympathetic nerve fibers of sleep apnea patients' leg muscles, and recorded their electrical activity during sleep. In contrast to healthy people, in whom there is reduced activity of the sympathetic nerves during sleep, the activity of the sleep apnea patients' neural fibers during sleep was twice as vigorous as when they were awake. Moreover, this heightened sympathetic activity in sleep apnea patients was not restricted to sleep, and even during wakefulness it was more vigorous than in healthy people.

We still have no complete explanation of how apneas during sleep cause more vigorous activity of the sympathetic system during the day. One possibility is that the frequent activation of the sympathetic system during sleep, resulting in elevated blood pressure, brings about a change in the way the baroreceptors, the neural sensors responsible for regulating blood pressure, work, or the way the chemoreceptors work, which is likely to heighten or reduce the activity of the sympathetic system in accordance with the changes that occur in blood gas levels.

The continuous activation of the sympathetic system is likely to have far-reaching clinical consequences, first and foremost among these being elevated blood pressure, which will bring in its wake other cardiovascular diseases.

Sclerosis—The Cardinal Sin

One of the broadest common denominators of cardiovascular disease is atherosclerosis. Far more deaths are attributed to atherosclerosis than to any other cause. In 1995 it was the cause of death of 685,000 Americans.

In a healthy person blood flows from the heart to all parts of the body through a ramified "pipeline," the total length of which is several kilometers. The arteries and arterioles through which blood flows can be likened to a many-branched irrigation system consisting of pipes of varying diameters that are sometimes blocked by an accumulation of scale and rust. Just like the garden pipeline, the blood vessels also sometimes restrict the flow, slowing it, due to residues that start blocking the arteries, until they are completely clogged. In 1904 the pathologist Felix Marchand coined the term "atherosclerosis" from two Greek words— *athero,* meaning "gruel," and *sklerosis,* "hardening"—and the name is eminently appropriate to the disease. Sclerosis is characterized by a gruel-like residue known as plaque that hardens on the artery walls, constricting their inner diameter and retarding the flow of blood. Like hypertension, atherosclerosis is often discovered only after the damage has been done. Unfortunately, in many cases the first indication that someone is suffering from atherosclerosis is a fatal heart attack or a stroke.

Until the 1970s there was a tendency to view atherosclerosis as the price paid by modern humans for their enthusiastic embrace of calorie- and fat-rich foods, a comfortable lifestyle without physical exercise, and smoking. The fact that rabbits fed with a cholesterol-rich diet developed atherosclerosis led to cholesterol becoming synonymous with all the causes of the disease, but we now know that this approach was too simplistic. Strange though it may seem, it appears that atherosclerosis begins to form at a very early age, perhaps even in infancy, and develops slowly over the years until the arterial blockage causes real damage. Today it is clear that atherosclerosis is not simply a disease of the convenient modern age, because examination of the arteries of Egyptian mummies has revealed it in some that were more than three thousand years old.

In the 1970s we gained a much clearer understanding of how the development of atherosclerosis really works. Since that time we no longer speak of the passive residue of fats on the artery walls, but of a complex and active process in which the cells of the immune system, the endothelial cells that cover the interior walls of the arteries, and fats carried by the bloodstream all take part. The new atherosclerosis theory is linked to the late Russell Ross of Washington University in Seattle. Ross began his career as a dentist but later specialized in experimental pathology, and he wrote his doctoral thesis on the healing of wounds. In the mid-1970s Ross propounded the hypothesis known today as the Ross-Glomset theory, according to which atherosclerosis is an uncontrolled inflammatory reaction of the arterial wall. In this process, the endothelial cells play a decisive role. The endothelium, or "lining," that covers the interior of the artery is a network of cells whose thickness is only a single cell, and it is this surface that comes into contact with the blood. The endothelial cells play a major role in controlling arterial blood flow. Through the secretion of nitric oxide (NO) molecules, the endothelial cells cause dilation of the arteries, thus enabling a greater flow of blood; a reduction in NO secretion causes constriction of the blood vessels, and consequently a reduction of blood flow and elevated blood pressure.

It was initially assumed that the endothelium was only the passive medium on which sclerosis was formed, and that it played no part in this formation. But today it is ascribed an active role in the sclerotic process. When any of the body's tissues are damaged as the result of an injury, a burn, or bacterial penetration, the body intensifies the flow of blood to the damaged tissue, and the immune system goes into action by sending white blood cells to the site. The white blood cells surround the affected area, and together with the cells of the injured tissue they work to repair the damage. A similar process takes place in the arteries, but the healing of damage to the artery wall is slower and takes longer, and it can end in a thickening of the interior wall of the artery, and even blockage. In other words, atherosclerosis.

The endothelial cells may be damaged for a number of reasons. Among these are high levels of cholesterol or the amino acid homocysteine, or from by-products of cigarette smoke, inflammatory factors, or because of a drop in blood oxygen saturation level that occurs every night, as it does in sleep apnea syndrome patients.

When the endothelial cells are damaged they produce special molecules, called adhesive molecules, on their surface. From the flow of blood over their surface they trap the white blood cells of the immune system, monocytes, and cells from the lymphocyte family. These cells adhere to

the endothelial cells like flies to a flypaper. Incidentally, adhesive molecules are not exclusive to endothelial cells: the body's cells also use them
to "trap" the white blood cells and "stick" them onto other wound sites.
But in atherosclerosis, the moment that the monocytes adhere to the
endothelial cells, the healing process spins out of control. The white
cells cause the destruction of the endothelial cells and the formation of
"foam cells" containing oxygenated lipids. Moreover, in a complex process, contact between the white and endothelial cells causes unregulated
growth in the smooth muscles on the artery wall. As a result, fatty strips
are formed on the artery walls that gradually thicken as layer upon layer
of "gruel," including cell residue and calcium, are laid on them.

In recent years the term "endothelial dysfunction" has increasingly
been used to describe a condition that might be called "pre-sclerotic,"
whereby damage is caused to the endothelial cells that disrupts their
function, albeit without a significant blockage of blood vessels. The function of the endothelial cells in controlling arterial blood flow is particularly impaired, because they do not produce sufficient quantities of NO,
and consequently the ability of the blood vessels to dilate is damaged. A
chronic condition of low NO levels and constricted arteries may cause
hypertension.

Apnea and Sclerosis Down Under

The first time I came across the idea that sleep apnea syndrome might be
connected to atherosclerosis was at a scientific conference in 1992 at a
small town with the exotic name of Palm Cove, on the Pacific coast of
northeastern Australia. The motto of the good citizens of Palm Cove,
which appears on shirts, cigarette lighters, mugs, and every other possible tourist memento, is "Down Under," the well-known nickname of
Australia and New Zealand. In Hebrew, "down under" is translated as
"world's end," and indeed beyond Palm Cove you can find only New
Zealand and Antarctica. The conference, organized by Colin Sullivan,
was attended by sleep researchers from all over the world who were interested in sleep apnea. Some of them immediately disappeared on hikes
through the dense rain forests, but there were also those who attended

all the lectures. Among the lecturers was Roger Dean, one of the most prominent researchers in the field of atherosclerosis, from the Sydney University Cardiac Research Unit.

Dean was invited to deliver a guest lecture on the disease and the exciting innovations connected with it, but not in the context of sleep apnea syndrome. He devoted a large part of his talk to free radicals and their importance in the sclerotic process. Free radicals are toxic oxygen molecules that are produced by the immune system cells for fighting off foreign invaders like bacteria. The body sometimes produces free radicals independently, especially under conditions in which there is a drop in the blood oxygen saturation level, and even more so when immediately after such a drop there is an increase in the blood oxygen level. Free radicals are attributed a key role in damage to the endothelial cells in the walls of the blood vessels that start the sclerotic process. At the conclusion of his lecture, Dean discussed the theoretical possibility that a recurring drop in the blood oxygen saturation level as a result of sleep apneas could cause increased production of free radicals, and consequently lead to damage to the endothelial cells and the onset of the sclerotic process.

Although my occupation as a sleep researcher is quite a long way away from atherosclerosis and its biochemical processes—almost as far as Haifa is from Palm Cove—Dean's lecture and the terminology he used were not entirely alien to me. My wife, Lena, wrote her doctoral thesis on inflammatory processes in aging, and the terms Dean used—free radicals, protein oxygenation, endothelial cells—were familiar from when Lena had done her doctoral research at the Technion Faculty of Biology. I suddenly realized that I didn't have to travel all the way to the end of the world to learn about the importance of sleep apnea syndrome in the development of atherosclerosis.

And so when I got back home from Down Under, we established a family research group in Haifa that focused on examining the possibility that a drop in the blood oxygen level in sleep apnea patients causes sclerotic processes and, as a result, cardiovascular diseases as well. Our team was joined by Larissa Dyugovskaya, an immunologist who had come to Israel in the big wave of emigration from the Soviet Union. Together, the combination of our biological, immunological, and clinical experience proved very successful.

Monocytes Out of Control

In atherosclerosis, as we have seen, white blood cells adhere to the endothelial cells with the help of adhesive molecules formed on the cells' surface. Accordingly, the presence of these molecules on the blood cells is the sign of an inflammatory condition. With the appearance of the adhesive cells, the body mobilizes the white cells and sends them to the site.

To investigate the connection with sleep apneas, Lena and Larissa isolated white blood cells in the blood of sleep apnea patients immediately after they awoke from a night's sleep, and then tested them for the presence of adhesive molecules. And indeed, on comparison with a group of healthy people, the sleep apnea patients' white blood cells were richer in adhesive molecules. Moreover, the sleep apnea patients' white blood cells were also "ready for battle," creating a greater number of free radicals than cells taken from the healthy subjects. To examine the significance of the nocturnal changes in the cells' function, Lena and Larissa added white blood cells from the sleep apnea patients and the control group to a human endothelial cell culture. About an hour later they examined the culture, which revealed that the white cells taken from the sleep apnea patients had gone into action and adhered to the endothelial cells. In contrast, the cells taken from the healthy people had not adhered to the endothelial cells in the culture. Interestingly, some patients were treated with continuous positive air pressure, or CPAP—essentially a mask attached to a compressor that pumps a regular flow of air through the nose during sleep, which prevents apneas—and these patients' cells also had not adhered, just like the healthy people's cells.

If the adhesion of the white blood cells to the endothelial cells in the petri dish indeed reflects what takes place in the patients' arteries, the experiment proved that every night sees vigorous sclerotic processes in the arteries of sleep apnea patients. Other researchers from Germany and Japan have also found an increase in the concentration of the adhesive molecules in the blood of sleep apnea patients.

Endothelial dysfunction, as described earlier, is a harbinger of atherosclerosis, and it was possible that we were also witnessing dysfunction in the endothelial cells of the sleep apnea patients. One way of testing the activity of these cells is by measurement of the level of NO, the molecule that distends the blood vessels, in the patients' blood. Studies conducted over the past two years have included analysis of blood samples taken from subjects immediately upon awakening in the morning. These have shown that in sleep apnea patients—who, importantly, did not suffer from any cardiovascular disease—the NO level is lower than it is in healthy people. CPAP treatment brought the NO level back to normal. In our laboratory we tested the NO level every hour through the night and found that it was significantly lower in sleep apnea patients than in people who were without the syndrome. Following CPAP treatment, the NO levels in the patients' blood showed a significant rise.

Another way of testing endothelial cell function is by examining the reaction of blood vessels to medication that enlarges their diameter through accelerating the secretion of NO molecules. When the reaction of the arteries of apnea patients who do not suffer from any other cardiovascular disease was examined, it became clear that the reaction of their blood vessels was less vigorous than it is in healthy people. In other words, sleep apnea syndrome is sufficient cause of a disruption in the dilation of the blood vessels.

These findings have far-reaching significance. If sleep apnea syndrome is indeed a risk factor for atherosclerosis that is slowly being built up night by night, then we must not wait for the appearance of such warning signs as severe daytime sleepiness or loud, intermittent snoring to start treating the syndrome. Treatment should begin as early as possible.

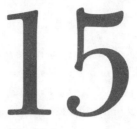

Death at an Early Age
and the Paradox of Old Age

In spite of their nocturnal battle for survival, sleep apnea patients do not usually die in their sleep as a result. The monitoring systems in their brains, which meticulously check the levels of carbon dioxide and oxygen in the blood, sense the approach of danger in good time and muster the assistance of the brain's wakefulness mechanisms. These power up before any physical damage can be done, awakening the sleeper and causing an immediate resumption of breathing. The awakening is so brief that it is not even recorded in the patient's memory. The brain, however, does remember these nocturnal awakenings, and they substantially influence levels of alertness and activity during the day.

Protecting the patient's life during sleep does not prevent cumulative damage to the heart and blood vessels as a result of frequent drops in blood oxygen levels and the repeated activation of the sympathetic nervous system. This damage, which accumulates over several years, increases the risk to the patient's life.

A comprehensive study on patient mortality necessitates continued monitoring of a large population, as well as gathering accurate information on medical condition and the circumstances of death, but this sort of information on sleep apnea patients is difficult to obtain. There is no methodical monitoring of patients in most laboratories, especially in a vast country like the United States, where mobility is great and it is difficult to keep track of people. Hence, most mortality studies involving sleep apnea syndrome have thus far relied on small groups of patients, which has made it impossible to draw definitive conclusions.

The first two studies of mortality in sleep apnea patients were carried out at Stanford and in Detroit. The Finnish sleep researcher Markku Partinen joined Stanford's sleep laboratory for a short time, and while there he and Christian Guilleminault investigated what had become of the two hundred or so sleep apnea patients who had been diagnosed at Stanford in the 1970s. Seventy-one of them had undergone tracheostomies, and 127 had been prescribed the more conservative treatment of reducing body weight. Fourteen patients had died in the five years since the examination; all of these, without exception, had been on the conservative treatment. Partinen and Guilleminault concluded that sleep apnea patients who remain untreated are at high risk of death, and tracheostomies significantly improve the life expectancy of sleep apnea patients.

The Detroit study was conducted by two doctors who are today ranked among the leading sleep researchers worldwide, Meir Kryger from Winnipeg, and Tom Roth, head of the Sleep Disorders and Research Center at Henry Ford Hospital in Detroit, and until recently the editor of *Sleep*. Although Kryger and Roth did not know each other in the early 1980s, they both participated in a study funded by the NIH to assess the effect of treating sleep apnea patients with oxygen during sleep. A number of years after collaborating from a distance, they met at a scientific conference in California and discovered that they had not only interests in common but similar family histories—both are children of Holocaust survivors who settled in North America. Kryger spent some years in Israel as a young boy before his parents emigrated to Canada.

When Kryger and Roth met in 1985, the sleep laboratory in Detroit was one of the leaders in diagnosis and treatment of sleep apnea patients in the United States. It kept its database current on all the patients who had been diagnosed there and the types of treatment prescribed for them—which in most cases included various surgical procedures, such as tracheostomy and widening the upper airways, or regimens based on weight reduction.

Their meeting in California led Kryger and Roth to a joint study on the mortality rate of sleep apnea patients. They located 385 of the 706 patients who had been examined in Detroit between 1978 and 1986, and found that 22 of them had died. Statistical analysis of the findings showed that the highest mortality risk was in patients younger than fifty who had suffered at least twenty apneas per hour. Tracheostomies or respiration during sleep significantly reduced mortality rates compared with people who had received no treatment at all or who had undergone surgical widening of the airways.

When Roth and Kryger's multiauthored paper was published in *Chest* in 1988, its list of authors was headed by an unknown researcher named J. He; no other paper in the field had been attributed to him before. The question of Dr. He's identity aroused curiosity among many sleep researchers, since position on the list of a scientific paper's authors is a very sensitive issue that can lead to tension and disputes, sometimes even ending long-term friendships in the process. In certain scientific fields the authors' names are listed alphabetically, but in most medical and life science publications the order of names is determined according to the relative contribution of each researcher. Most of the disputes between research partners are over the first and last places on the list. The researcher who contributed most significantly to the study appears first, and the last name is usually the head of the research group, or the senior researcher of the group that led the study.

Jiang He, it turned out, was a young doctor from China who had appeared one morning in Meir Kryger's office in Winnipeg and told him excitedly that the Chinese government had sent him for further studies at his laboratory, and here he was, raring to go. Although Kryger had been completely unaware that a doctor from China was about to start working at his laboratory, he assumed that the arrangements had been made "upstairs," at the university, and welcomed him. As it happened, He was a talented researcher, and Kryger assigned him to the team researching mortality in sleep apnea patients. He proceeded to spend day and night gathering data, processing it, and preparing it for publication, emerging by his efforts as the leading member of the team. One day, about six months later, after the paper had been submitted for publication, He came into Kryger's office and told him shamefacedly that there had been a terrible mistake. He had been working in the wrong laboratory; he had actually been sent on a study program in physiology, not sleep research. Surprised, Kryger wished him every success in his new field.

Other studies supported the Detroit finding that younger sleep apnea patients were at the highest risk for mortality. In 1984, Eva Lindberg and her colleagues had assessed the prevalence of complaints of chronic snoring, daytime sleepiness, and other sleep disorders in 3,100 residents of the city of Uppsala in Sweden. Ten years later, Lindberg returned to find out what had become of Uppsala's residents, especially the sleepy ones and the snorers among them, and she found that 213 of them had died. When the association between the deaths and the complaints recorded in 1984 was examined, it showed that mortality among snorers and sleepy people sixty and older was identical to that of the rest of the population. But in the age group between thirty and fifty, the risk for death among the snorers and the sleepy ones was seven times higher than in people who had not complained of snoring or sleepiness.

Findings on mortality of sleep apnea patients at the Technion's sleep laboratory also pointed in the same direction. In 1995, we studied mortality rates among the 1,607 people who had been examined at our laboratories between 1976 and 1988. Fifty-seven of the patients had died, half of them from causes related to heart disease, the blood vessels, and the respiratory system. We found that the highest risk for mortality was in young patients, thirty to fifty years old; among patients older than fifty there was no excess mortality in comparison with the general Israeli population.

We have recently completed a similar study, but this time using a much larger population of patients. Between 1985 and 2000, approximately 35,000 people were examined at the Technion's sleep laboratories in Haifa, Jerusalem, Tel Aviv, and Holon. Some 80 percent of them were diagnosed with sleep apnea syndrome. Using the database of the Ministry of Interior's Population Registry, we investigated what had become of every patient. We found that 1,144 of them had died by 2000, and in half of them either cardiovascular or respiratory disease was the cause of death. When we adjusted for age and gender, in sleep apnea patients aged twenty to fifty the mortality rate was significantly higher than in the general population, for both women and men. In contrast, in older sleep apnea patients, people over fifty, the mortality rate was no different than in the general population, in both men and women—the same results as we had earlier found in a much smaller population.

How can these findings be interpreted?

The first possible explanation is that breathing disorders during sleep in the elderly may not be as severe as in the young; hence, they have no clinical significance. As we have seen, several studies indicate that sleep breathing disorders are highly prevalent among the elderly, and are usually unrelated to complaints about quality of sleep or daytime sleepiness. But, as far as the data from the Technion's sleep laboratory showed, comparison of the syndrome's severity in young and elderly sleep apnea patients who died did not indicate significant variances in the syndrome's severity in terms of the number of apneas per hour, or drops in blood oxygen levels.

A second possibility is that the elderly people with sleep apnea syndrome may represent a unique group of "survivors." Similar paradoxical findings have also been reported for cholesterol levels and hypertension. In contrast to young people and the middle-aged, for whom high cholesterol is a risk factor for mortality, it is not for those over seventy. On the contrary, a ten-year follow-up study of elderly patients eighty-five and older revealed an inverse relation between blood cholesterol concentrations and mortality—in their cases, the lower the concentration of cholesterol, the higher the risk for mortality, both in women and in men. Similar findings have also been reported concerning hypertension.

There is, however, a third possibility—one that, although still pure conjecture, is fascinating and kindles the imagination. In the previous chapter we saw the evidence that damage to the cardiovascular system in sleep apnea patients begins even on the first night of disrupted breathing, with this damage accumulating over several years. It is possible that, with a slow process of cumulative damage, some sleep apnea patients may adapt to the syndrome, which could provide them with protection against cardiovascular disease. New findings from our laboratory and others indicate that the adaptation process in sleep apnea patients is not merely theoretical conjecture.

Every drop in blood oxygen levels is highly consequential to the survivability of an organism, so much so that evolution has created special sensory mechanisms to monitor oxygen levels in the body's tissue in order to enable protective action in every event of deviation from the norm. As soon as the sensors detect a deviation, special protein-producing genes are activated. The protein produced in this way is called vascular endothelial growth factor (VEGF), and its role is to grow new blood vessels. The new blood vessels improve blood supply to the tissue, thus compensating for the drop in oxygen. For example, it has been found that there is an increase in VEGF protein concentration in the cardiac cells after a heart attack caused by blockage of blood supply to the cardiac muscle. Growth of new blood vessels around the heart protects it from possible damage caused by the drop in blood supply. Recently, it has even been suggested that cardiac atherosclerosis patients should be treated with genes that control production of the protein. People differ from one another, probably genetically, in their ability to produce the VEGF protein in response to a drop in oxygen levels. Some respond vigorously in such circumstances and produce large quantities of VEGF, whereas others are insensitive to changes in oxygen levels. Narrowing of the arteries in those who respond to drops in oxygen levels by producing the VEGF protein leads to increased growth of new blood vessels around the heart. In people who are insensitive to drops in oxygen levels, no new blood vessels are formed. Consequently, people who respond by producing new blood vessels have better protection against heart attacks.

Recently we found, as did other research groups from Japan, Germany, and the United States, that in some cases nocturnal drops in blood oxygen levels in sleep apnea patients lead to a rise in concentration of the VEGF protein. Improving patients' blood oxygen levels leads to a drop in concentration of the protein in their blood. It is possible, therefore, that in response to a drop in blood oxygen levels some people are able to increase production of the protein that accelerates growth of new blood vessels. As a result, a network of blood vessels forms around their heart, ensuring regular blood supply to the cardiac muscle, thus protecting the patient from the destructive consequences of sclerosis. It may be that these people live longer than those who do not have this type of "safety net."

As I have said, of course, this is still mere conjecture. To prove it, we need to investigate whether sleep apnea patients who have reached old age have more blood vessels around their hearts than their healthy peers. Whatever the explanation, something is helping certain older sleep apnea patients to adapt to the syndrome, even as the syndrome is contributing to the risk of mortality for those who are still in their younger years. In any case, treatment of the syndrome's causes to prevent the occurrence of the nightly apneas, and the constant blood oxygen depletion associated with them, is the only effective means of reducing those added mortality risks.

16

Treatments for Sleep Apnea Syndrome

A wide gap exists between the great ease with which sleep apnea syndrome can be diagnosed and the equally great difficulty in finding an effective treatment for it. This is not because effective treatments are lacking, but rather because of the discomfort they impose on patients.

A good example is weight reduction. There is no doubt that losing weight improves the condition of the sleepy patient, as ample evidence has shown beginning with the first Pickwickians in the nineteenth century. Modern studies reveal that a reduction of 10 to 20 percent of body weight results in a 50 percent decrease in the number of apneas during sleep. The solution is simple: "all" the patient has to do is lose weight. Disappointingly, however, this solution is not at all simple and is far from easy.

The heavier patients are, the harder it is for them to lose weight by conventional means. The majority of people who suffer from obesity spend their lives desperately searching for ways of losing weight. There is no dieting method they haven't tried and no slimming expert they haven't consulted. Most people who do lose weight find that their success is short-lived. Soon after the conclusion of an apparently successful treatment, a massive weight increase takes place, often raising the person's weight above what it had been in the first place. In most cases the difficulty is not just in losing weight but in maintaining the new weight. The more accepted methods of losing weight include behavioral therapy designed to change eating habits and habits connected with physical exercise, a "killer" diet of four hundred to eight hundred calories per day, or prescription of appetite suppressants.

Behavioral therapy is usually in the form of group therapy—various kinds of weight-watcher groups that meet on a regular basis and share experiences as members try to harness their appetites. The aim of the meetings is to provide the participants with positive reinforcement for every step they take, even the tiniest, toward losing weight. These programs are mainly suitable for people with Grade 1 obesity, and in such people it is hard to find any who have managed to lose more than fifteen kilograms even after a year or more of therapy. Limiting daily intake to four hundred to eight hundred calories for a limited time is very effective, but in most cases the weight will return to its previous levels, and will even pass them. Apart from dieting, there are no wonder drugs for losing weight. Over the past decade numerous appetite suppressants have been abandoned because of undesirable side effects. In 1997, two leading appetite suppressants, Redux and Fen-Fen, were removed from drugstore shelves after it became clear that they were liable to cause heart valve damage.

For the majority of obese people, especially those with Grades 2 and 3 obesity, the only chance for breaking the vicious circle of rising and falling weight is a procedure called bariatric surgery, or stomach reduction. The basic premise is simple: reducing the stomach's volume, using surgery to create a "pocket" in the stomach that limits intake to four hundred to six hundred calories per day. This severe restriction causes a rapid loss of body weight—up to twenty or twenty-five kilograms in the first three months after the operation. Within six months the expected weight loss is 40–50 percent of body weight. The weight loss gradually diminishes and stops after about eighteen months, when body weight stabilizes at 60–75 percent less than the starting weight. During this period the patient must get used to new eating habits and far smaller quantities of food than accustomed. For many years these procedures were the subject of contentious debates, but in sleep apnea patients they have been a resounding success.

Professor Ilan Charuzi was among the first surgeons in Israel to spe-

cialize in stomach reduction procedures when he was head of the surgical department at the Soroka Medical Center in Beersheba. I first met him
at an Israeli Surgical Society conference in Haifa in 1982, which I attended especially to hear his lecture on the surgical procedure for extremely obese people. My experiences with sleep apnea in such patients
had made it clear that treatment would not work for them if it did not
adopt a drastic approach. After the lecture I buttonholed Charuzi and
told him about the relationship between obesity and sleep apnea syndrome and proposed that he examine the effect of massive weight reduction through surgery on the sleep respiratory function on these patients.
His response was direct and immediate: "I do the largest number of surgical procedures on obese people in Israel. Let's study this together." The
result was a ten-year series of joint Beersheba-Haifa studies on the sleep
of the very obese before and after the stomach reduction procedure.

The first thing we found was that sleep apnea syndrome is far more
prevalent among the very obese than in the general population. One in
every three people who applied for surgery because of obesity suffered
from the syndrome, and moreover in most cases the syndrome was very
severe. In both populations, the regular and the obese, the syndrome's
prevalence among men was greater than among women, and it generally
appeared in the thirty-five-plus age group. The stomach reduction procedure brought about dramatic changes, in both the patient's weight and
the quality of sleep. A laboratory follow-up recording of the sleep of
people who had undergone the surgery showed that all those who lost
weight improved their sleep respiratory function beyond recognition.
To our surprise, in many cases the sleep breathing disorder disappeared
completely, and in some cases the disturbances in heart rhythms during
sleep also disappeared and blood pressure fell. The improvement was so
dramatic that in one tracheostomy case we were able to close the surgical opening.

It is interesting to note that the total disappearance of apneas during sleep was common to different people of different weights. There
were cases in which only a moderate weight reduction—of 20 kilograms,
from 140 to 120—was sufficient to improve the quality of breathing during sleep, while in others of the same weight no improvement was evi-

dent until they lost 40–50 kilograms. It appears that every person has a particular weight threshold beyond which breathing during sleep is impaired.

Our articles on the subject were published in the leading scientific journals, but the medical community did not go out of its way to adopt the surgical approach for sleep apnea syndrome; in fact, there was also some opposition to it. At one of the first medical conferences devoted to sleep apnea syndrome held in Milan, Charuzi described the success of surgery in weight reduction, citing one extraordinarily obese patient as an example. The patient had come to the Technion Sleep Laboratory from Brussels, weighed in at 200 kilograms, and spent most of his day sleeping. On a number of occasions he had fallen asleep in dangerous situations that had resulted in injury. His sleep recordings showed a record number of apneas, more than a hundred per hour. In the summarizing talk following the examination, we made it clear that there was no likelihood of curing his apneas during sleep without him losing more than half his body weight. Like most extremely obese patients, this man had undergone countless dietetic and other treatments aimed at reducing his weight, but to no avail. So we suggested that he travel to Beersheba and meet with Professor Charuzi to examine the possibility of undergoing the stomach reduction procedure. The patient accepted our proposal, underwent the surgery, and the results were dramatic.

Before our very eyes the patient shed dozens of kilograms in a very short time. To document the process, we conducted further sleep recordings as his weight dropped to 160, 120, and 100 kilograms. The improvement in his sleep increased as his body weight decreased, and when it reached 100 kilograms, half his original weight, the sleep apnea syndrome disappeared completely. He slept through the whole night as peacefully as a babe, with no breathing disorders at all. Together with his loss of weight, his daytime sleepiness also disappeared, and there were no further complaints about his stentorian snoring.

It was obviously a dramatic case, but to our surprise the audience of sleep apnea specialists in Milan did not greet our presentation with cries of amazement. Quite the contrary. The questions they asked were skeptical, and to a great extent hectoring: "Don't you feel that the stomach reduction procedure is too aggressive and dangerous for treating sleep apnea syndrome?" "Aren't you putting these patients at risk with this operation?" "What is the percentage of mortality in these procedures?" and so on. Charuzi, angry and upset, answered his critics with typical Israeli directness: "The fact that all our patients are still our close friends after the surgery is sufficient evidence of the extent to which we have changed their lives." And indeed, the lives of the majority of the post-operative patients were changed beyond recognition. In Israel today, some 1,500 stomach reduction procedures are done each year, and our accumulated experience shows that approximately two-thirds of the patients manage to significantly reduce their weight, while the other third "overcome" the pocket in their stomach and regain the lost weight.

It should be emphasized, however, that this is not a miracle cure. As with any surgical procedure, the possibility of complications and even failure always exists. The American Society for Bariatric Surgery recommends the procedure for patients who are younger than forty years of age and have a BMI of at least 40. Moreover, anyone who chooses the operation must first understand that it will change his or her life drastically, particularly with regard to eating habits. But the extremely obese person who suffocates during sleep night after night is also at high risk for cardiovascular disease and death, and in such cases the possible risks of surgery are likely to seem comparatively small.

Can we conclude from the results of stomach reduction procedures that obesity was the only reason these patients suffered from sleep apnea syndrome? Not at all. A follow-up ten years after patients underwent the procedure and lost a great deal of weight shows that a small group was still burdened with sleep disorders, even though their body weight had not increased.

From Scalpel to Laser

Tracheostomy was the first treatment to completely and immediately resolve the problem of sleep apnea syndrome. The procedure itself has a long and rich history. Galen mentioned it some two thousand years ago,

when he wrote that opening the upper section of the windpipe is recommended only if the patient suffocates and is on the verge of dying. In
medieval times, tracheostomy was referred to with awe. There was no
other operation that could save a person from death, and certainly not in
such a dramatic fashion. Hieronymus Fabricius of Venice declared in his
seventeenth-century work *Operationes Chirurigicae:* "There is no operation like the tracheostomy for adding to the physician's honor and plac-
ing him next to the gods."

Exactly how many sleep apnea patients have been treated with tracheostomy is unknown, but it is not many, in spite of the procedure's effectiveness. Of the hundreds of patients diagnosed at our Haifa and Tel
Aviv laboratories in the late 1970s and early 1980s, perhaps ten were
treated in this way, and in each case the syndrome posed a very real danger to the patient's life. The main reason for the paucity of operations
was that the majority of the patients were repelled by the idea of having
a stoma in their throat. In addition to the esthetic aspect, tracheostomy
can be accompanied by troublesome side effects, such as infection of the
stoma, fluid accumulation, and speech difficulties.

For patients who are not prepared to undergo tracheostomy, other
approaches try to prevent upper airway blockage by widening the airways. Once it became clear that many patients viewed tracheostomy as
far too drastic a treatment for sleep disordered breathing, other surgical
procedures, some simple and some complex, were developed. The first
attempts were designed to widen the nasal airways, the assumption
being that if they are particularly narrow, the act of breathing creates a
greater negative pressure in the thorax, thus causing the collapse of the
pharynx. This assumption gained further credence when it became clear
that a misshapen nasal septum—a common cause of narrowed nasal airways—is extremely prevalent in sleep apnea syndrome patients. Consequently, a great many surgical procedures to correct this fault were conducted on sleep apnea patients, but it quickly became clear that the
improvement in their sleep was only temporary. Although the septum
was straightened and the patients reported a vast improvement in their
breathing and sleep, examinations in the sleep laboratory revealed that
the breathing disorders had not lessened.

The results of tonsillectomies in adult patients were also disappointing. In children, as we have seen, tonsillectomy is something of a miracle treatment, but in adults the procedure brought only temporary relief of sleep breathing disorders. In light of these failures, it became clear that a more significant widening of the airways was called for, and this conclusion led to a new surgical procedure with a name as convoluted as the airways themselves: uvulopalatopharyngeal plastic surgery, or UPPP. The name comes from the areas to which the surgeon's scalpel is applied: the uvula, the soft palate, and the pharynx. The basic idea is not much different from that of tonsillectomy or straightening the nasal septum. In order to reduce the risk of pharyngeal collapse during sleep, all the soft tissue likely to collapse and obstruct the airways is removed. From the oral cavity the surgeon takes the remains of the tonsils, the atrophied and excess tissues from the soft palate, and even the uvula, that small protuberance that peeks out from the oral cavity when we open our mouth in front of a mirror.

To this day in extensive areas of Africa, it is common practice to remove the uvula in infancy to prevent throat infections and various other illnesses. This custom was also prevalent among the Jews of Ethiopia. We have no information on the possibility that removing the uvula in infancy provides protection against sleep disordered breathing in adulthood.

The second half of the 1980s saw a rise in the popularity of UPPP, partly as a result of the introduction of laser surgery, which causes less pain during and after the operation than traditional surgery with a scalpel. A UPPP operation that is done with a laser is called laser-assisted uvulopalatoplasty, or LAUP, and is usually done in a doctor's office under local anesthetic, in two to four appointments. Using the laser the surgeon removes the excess tissue from the pharynx and oral cavity and excises the uvula. UPPP surgery in the United States was pioneered by Shiro Fujita of Detroit, who published the first report in English on it in 1984, and since then more than two hundred articles on the procedure and its results have appeared. Interestingly, this procedure was practiced in Japan for several years before it was introduced in the West.

The first reports on the results of the procedure were encouraging, especially when it was not followed by sleep laboratory tests and its success was measured only by the subjective report of the patient. But close scrutiny of the articles, from the very first one, shows that not all the patients responded to the procedure in the same way. There were some for whom the procedure indeed brought about a significant change in respiratory function during sleep, but in others no change took place at all. The variations in the success rates of different surgeons were influenced by a number of factors, including the type of patient operated on, whether scalpel or laser technique was used, the degree of the surgeon's aggressiveness, whether the surgeon removed only the excess tissue or also the entire uvula, and, most important of all, how the surgeon defined surgical success.

It appeared that the definition of surgical success was extremely flexible. There were those who considered the procedure successful if a patient reported sleeping better, snoring less, and feeling more alert during the day. But others relied on a post-operative sleep laboratory examination and defined success as at least a 50 percent reduction in the number of apneas during sleep. The strictest definitions ruled the operation a success only when the number of apneas dropped to below ten per hour, the most common criterion for defining sleep apnea syndrome.

I remember a scientific conference on sleep apnea, held in Bordeaux, at which a French surgeon presented an amazing picture of surgical successes using UPPP. He said that almost 100 percent of his patients made a full recovery from the syndrome. When one of the skeptics in the audience asked him how he determined that the patients had recovered from sleep disordered breathing, his laconic reply was, "I asked them." It turned out that the surgeon had not taken the trouble to check whether any change had taken place in his patients' weight after the operation, a most significant fact, as many patients who undergo UPPP surgery lose weight because of difficulty in swallowing. Small wonder, then, that these patients reported an improvement in their condition. In addition, marketing efforts portray the procedure as a trivial affair in which there is almost no discomfort, but many patients reported severe pain, especially during the first few days after the operation. The pain, too, contributed to the enforced diet and indirectly to the patients' much-improved condition. But as the surgical scars healed, the patients' weight returned to what it was before, as did the sleep breathing disorders, sleepiness, and snoring. Follow-ups conducted some two years after the operation showed that fewer than half of the patients reported any improvement in their condition.

Another recent innovation in the field of pharyngeal surgery as a sleep apnea treatment is the use of microwaves to shrink the soft tissue. Needles inserted into the nasal cavities and the pharyngeal area radiate microwaves, which cause vaporization of part of the tissue and some local cauterization, followed by shrinking of the tissue during the recovery period. This procedure is also done under local anesthetic at the doctor's office. Although there is still not a great deal of accumulated experience in the use of microwave radiation, according to the results reported so far the method is particularly suitable for snorers and only mild cases of sleep apnea. In addition, it appears that the treatment has to be repeated every few months because of recurring tissue thickening in the cauterized area.

More significant success in treating sleep apnea has been achieved using maxillary-mandibular advancement, a surgical procedure that tries to make a radical change in a patient's facial structure. The lower and upper jaws are shifted from their places and moved forward, which leaves a greater space for airflow in the area of the pharynx and oral cavity, thus preventing the nocturnal blockage. These procedures are done under general anesthetic on patients who suffer from severe sleep apnea syndrome. According to some reports, the success rate of these procedures reaches over 90 percent.

What's a Dentist Doing in the Sleep Laboratory?

Charles F. Samelson, a Chicago psychiatrist and chronic snorer who bothered his family with his loud snoring, and who completely recoiled from surgery, endeavored to find an original solution to his problem. He built a plastic device that looked something like a basketball player's mouth guard, with an opening that held his tongue and kept it from falling backward while he was asleep. When Samelson first showed me his "tongue holder" many years ago, my first thought was, What happens if the tongue can't be released in the morning? Apparently, the same thought occurred to many other people, for Samelson's invention did not gain a large number of supporters. But he was not the first to think about a mechanical device that would widen the airways during sleep.

The first attempts at widening the airways using dental appliances were made in the 1930s, and not in the context of sleep apnea. Pierre Rubin, a French pediatrician, treated children born without a lower jaw or with a degenerated jaw. The children's facial disfigurement caused them to suffocate when lying on their backs because there was nothing to stop the tongue from falling backward and blocking the pharynx. To prevent this, Rubin used dental appliances that enabled the children to sleep safely. A degenerated lower jaw that causes breathing difficulty when lying on the back is known today as Pierre Rubin syndrome. Meir Ewart and his colleagues from the Treise Neurological Hospital in Germany adopted Rubin's approach for treating sleep apnea patients. At the seventh conference of the European Sleep Research Society, held in 1984, they presented for the first time their dental appliance for the lower jaw; its purpose was to bring the jaw forward, thus widening the airways of sleep apnea patients. Examination of patients who slept wearing a dental appliance showed an improvement in their breathing while asleep in comparison to their sleep without it. Since then the field of sleep disorders has been opened to another professional group, the dental surgeons, especially in North America, and the sphere of dental appliances has flourished.

The idea behind all dental appliances is the same: bringing the lower jaw and tongue forward, thus widening the airway. The appliances differ in the physical attributes of the materials from which they are made and the extent to which they bring the jaw forward. There are permanent appliances that bring the jaw forward by only three or four millimeters, while others bring it forward by eight millimeters and in some cases by even more. Treatment with a dental appliance is usually suitable for mild or moderate cases or for patients who refuse any other treatment.

Like many other sleep researchers, I had some initial doubts about the efficacy of this treatment. But the stubbornness of a close friend who used a dental appliance for many years, and who also introduced me to Professor Glenn Clark of the UCLA School of Dentistry, made me change my mind. L.R. was among the first sleep apnea patients in the world to be treated nightly with a dental appliance. As a result of our friendship, he insisted that I meet Clark, who had made his appliance, and even suggested that Clark and the Technion Sleep Laboratory conduct a joint study on the appliance's effectiveness. Thus a project was born that bridged almost sixty-five hundred miles between Los Angeles and Haifa. Once Clark had come to Israel and instructed our colleagues from the oral and maxillofacial surgery department at the Rambam Medical Center in preparing the dental appliance molds, the molds were sent to Los Angeles where the appliances were built. At the sleep laboratory we examined sleep apnea patients before and after the dental appliance treatment. The research results verified L.R.'s claim that the appliance did indeed improve respiratory function during sleep, particularly for patients with mild to moderate forms of the syndrome.

Recent years have seen numerous studies proving the efficacy of treatment with dental appliances, and their use has become more and more common. But like other treatment methods that became popular overnight, the dental appliance has some drawbacks. First, the efficacy of many of the appliances constantly being offered to patients has not been tested. Some researchers have estimated that, of the twenty-five appliances currently in use, only eleven have been reliably studied. Dental appliances are also fitted to patients without a sleep examination and without any documentation of sleep disorder. In some cases it is enough for a patient to mention a habit of snoring loudly for the dentist to suggest fitting a dental appliance to solve the problem. And whether it actually works is not tested in most patients; in only 20 percent of people treated with a dental appliance is any kind of efficacy evaluation of the treatment undertaken.

And, finally, we do not have sufficient information on all the phenomena associated with the treatment, especially over a long period. Here and there we have seen reports of increased salivation, a feeling of discomfort in the teeth, and jaw joint pains, but this information is purely preliminary. There is still a need to investigate whether prolonged use of a dental appliance is likely to change the patient's occlusion (the fit of the

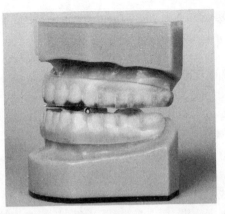

A dental device for sleep apnea treatment
that moves the lower jaw forward

teeth when the jaws are closed) and cause either loosening of the teeth or
pain in the jaw joints. In any event, patients considering a dental appliance should consult a dentist who is in close contact with a sleep laboratory to ensure that the dentist is at least informed about sleep disorders
and that the treatment's efficacy is suitably examined. Patients should
also request full information on the type of appliance to be fitted and on
the efficacy tests that have been conducted for it.

How About a Breathing Pill?

The dream of numerous sleep apnea patients is to swallow a pill every
night before bed that will, as if by the wave of a magic wand, make snoring and apneas vanish. But success in the search for a miracle pill has so
far been elusive. A great number of drugs for treating sleep apnea have
been tried, most of which were based on random clinical observations,
and not one has been found effective. Because the incidence of sleep
apnea syndrome is lower in women of childbearing age than in meno-
pausal women, for example, and because the female hormone progesterone stimulates the respiratory center, there was an assumption that
perhaps sleep disorders in men could be treated with progesterone. Disappointingly, the improvement in respiratory function during sleep was

insignificant, especially in relation to the side effects of administering a female hormone to men. In the early 1980s, when we tried treating a small number of patients with progesterone, they came back to the laboratory a few days later complaining that the treatment had robbed them of "the only pleasure left to them," their sex life, and the negligible improvement in their sleep was no compensation. Other treatments, using a similar logic, have also tried using thyroxine, the hormone secreted by the thyroid gland, but this too proved to be a disappointment.

Stimulating the respiratory center has also been the object of other drug treatments, particularly theophylline and acetozolamide. Acetozolamide causes metabolic acidosis that stimulates the respiratory system. It was found that this treatment improved sleep respiratory function in people suffering from central apneas, but not obstructive and mixed episodes. Moreover, in a number of cases the treatment even exacerbated the condition of patients with obstructive problems. Theophylline, which is mainly used to treat asthmatics, operates through an unknown mechanism, but it is assumed that it activates the respiratory center by increasing the metabolic rate or intensifying the action of the respiratory muscles. As with acetozolamide, it mainly improved the sleep respiratory function of people afflicted by either central events or periodic breathing, but not in cases of obstruction. In addition, together with the improvement in sleep respiratory function, theophylline caused disruption of the sleep pattern itself, thus impairing its efficacy. As only a small number of sleep apnea patients suffer from central apneas, these two drugs do not provide a solution to the problem of the lion's share of patients.

Psychotropic drugs that affect the central nervous system are usually used to treat excessive sleepiness, particularly in narcoleptics. Once it became clear that a narcoleptic patient who also suffered from sleep apnea syndrome had been successfully treated with the psychotropic drug protryptyline, it was tried on sleep apnea syndrome patients. The drug brought about a certain improvement in the patients' breathing, but only indirectly. As protryptyline shortened REM sleep, the sleep stage in which the longest apneas take place, the drug reduced the number of long apneas. Protryptyline can therefore be successfully used in the treatment of patients who have apneas only during REM sleep.

In summing up everything known so far about pharmacological

treatment of sleep breathing suspensions, we may say that all the attempts have been casual and coincidental, and almost all of them were disappointing. None of the pharmacological experiments professed to treat the source of the nocturnal problem, blockage of the upper airways. All of them tried to either stimulate the respiratory center into more vigorous activity or to reduce the duration of sleep in which the most severe apneas appeared.

But the drug company that can crack the neurochemical code for control of the muscles that collapse during sleep, and develop a wonder pill to prevent that collapse, will surely have a success on its hands to rival Pfizer's for its development of Viagra to counter impotence.

The Tennis Ball Method

In certain cases a change of habit may contribute to enhancing sleep respiratory function. For example, many patients are unaware that drinking alcoholic beverages before going to sleep exacerbates sleep respiratory disorders, because alcohol depresses respiratory activity. A number of studies have shown that alcohol also contributes to sleep apnea syndrome, especially the nightly drop in the blood oxygen level. Sleeping pills have a similar effect as most of them depress respiratory function. Patients unaware that the source of their sleep disorders is in the disruption of respiratory activity during sleep, and who use sleeping pills, are unintentionally exacerbating their condition. Under the influence of sleeping pills, the apneas become more prolonged, and consequently the drop in blood oxygen level is increased. Accordingly, a change in the habit of imbibing alcoholic drinks and taking sleeping pills is likely, to a certain extent, to improve respiratory function during sleep.

But the most efficient behavioral change is in sleeping posture. A large number of studies have shown that sleeping on the back exacerbates sleep apneas; furthermore, some people experience sleep apneas only when lying on their backs. There is a simple method for avoiding sleeping on the back: sew a pocket into the back of the pajama jacket or nightgown and put a tennis ball in it. Turning onto the back causes the ball to bother the patient, who will then turn onto his or her side.

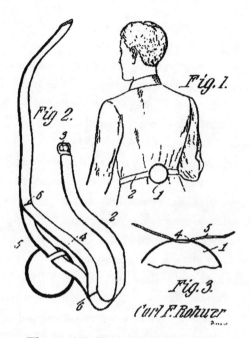

The tennis ball method for preventing
snoring, from a U.S. patent circa 1900

Rosalind Cartwright, a veteran American sleep researcher, and
Arieh Oksenberg of the Loewenstein Hospital Sleep Laboratory in Israel,
are two of the tennis ball method's greatest proponents. According to
comparative data, breathing disorders when lying on the back are worse
than in any other sleeping position. This is because of changes in the collapse threshold of the upper airways when lying on the back, but there are
other consequences as well. When sleep apnea patients are treated with
continuous positive air pressure, those who sleep on their backs need a
higher treatment pressure. Preventing sleeping on the back is effective
for patients with a mild or moderate form of the syndrome, but it has no
significant effect on those who have a severe form of the syndrome.

The sleep examination findings in astronauts who showed a dramatic improvement in sleep respiratory function in space suggest the
possibility of treating sleep respiratory disorders by neutralizing the
force of gravity. Perhaps treatment of this kind, currently only in the
realm of science fiction, will become reality within the next few years.

Electrical Stimulation to Prevent Apneas

Another possible way of correcting the disruption in the neural control of the muscles that widen the upper airways is by external electrical stimulation. The first report on a therapeutic experiment of this kind in patients with sleep apnea syndrome was published in 1989, by Hiroshi Miki and his colleagues from Tohoku University in Sendai, Japan. They reported that electrical stimulation, provided by electrodes placed under the chin of six sleep apnea patients, reduced the number of apneas and brought about a great improvement in the quality of their sleep. According to their report, the electrical stimulus, which was applied at the beginning of each apnea, did not cause any disruption in the continuity of sleep. These findings showed great promise, but attempts to verify them in further studies have met with no success.

Other experiments in electrical stimulation have tried using electrodes in the form of tiny needles inserted directly into the lingual, or tongue, muscles, but these have had mixed results. In some of them, electrical stimulation indeed reduced the number of apneas and lessened the severity of the syndrome, whereas in others it had almost no effect on the sleep apneas. Moreover, in many cases the electrical stimulus caused awakening from sleep. Peter Herman and his colleagues at Phillips University in Marbourg, Germany, and Allan Schwartz and his colleagues from Johns Hopkins University in Baltimore, have accumulated vast experience in applying electrical stimulation to both the lingual nerves and the lingual muscles. They argue that the precise anatomical location where stimulus is applied matters greatly: stimulation in one place will cause increased airflow, and in another, adjacent location it is liable to produce the opposite effect.

Christian Guilleminault and his colleagues tested one of the first commercial versions of an electrical appliance for stimulation of the lingual muscles in 1995, and they summed up their findings by saying, "there is currently no support for the claim that electrical stimulus is an efficacious treatment for sleep apnea syndrome." Following this judgment, in the second half of the 1990s very few studies on electrical stimulation in sleep apnea syndrome patients were conducted. Initial enthusiasm gave way to disappointment, and it is almost certain that the failures disheartened many, including the commercial companies that might have developed electrical stimulus instruments. Even so, electrical stimulation treatment has potential for the future. The development of miniaturized electrical stimulators of the kind used for intracerebral stimulation in Parkinson's disease patients, or for controlling incontinence in the chronically ill, promises that the day is not far off when we will be able to implant miniaturized stimulator units into the lingual muscles to prevent the tongue from falling backward during sleep.

17

Sleeping Under Pressure—
The Big Promise

About ten years ago, I traveled to Sydney, Australia, for a scientific conference on sleep apnea syndrome. When I landed at the airport, I noticed a strange phenomenon. Wherever I looked there were people wearing red plastic noses, like circus clowns. At first I assumed that I had happened upon some kind of local carnival, but there didn't seem to be any other fancy dress involved. It turned out that I had arrived on Red Nose Day, which marks the Australian national fundraising drive for the fight against crib death.

In addition to heightening awareness of crib death, Australia has made a considerable contribution to sleep apnea patients. Innumerable people with sleep apnea owe their gratitude to an Australian, Colin Sullivan. In 1982, Sullivan discovered the most effective treatment for sleep apnea syndrome—continuous positive air pressure, or CPAP.

Sullivan was infected by the sleep research bug early in his career. After completing his medical studies and specializing in respiratory medicine, Sullivan returned to the University of Sydney in 1972 for his doctoral studies under the tutelage of the physiologist David Read, who was researching the respiratory control mechanism. Sullivan's doctoral thesis was on the role played in respiratory control by reflexes originating from sensors that discern the degree of tension in the lung walls. As Sullivan had accumulated research experience during his undergraduate studies, and was blessed with a magic touch in all things technical, he became the driving force in establishing the David Read Laboratory for respiratory control. Shortly afterward, David Henderson-Smart, who researched respiratory function in the sleep of infants, and Michael Hensley, who had developed a clinical test to assess respiratory response to falling levels of oxygen concentration in humans, joined the team.

The group invested considerable research in efforts to gain insight into the causes of crib death. There is great interest in the syndrome in Australia, but Read had a personal stake in the research. One of his closest friend's babies was found unconscious in his sleep; the child survived, but with brain damage. Like many others, Read presumed that crib death was caused by a prolonged apnea. His research group became involved in sleep apnea in adults by chance. One of the patients at the Royal Prince Alfred Hospital in Sydney was well known to all the respiratory medicine interns. Albie C. was an overweight truck driver who was also a heavy drinker and smoker. Everybody knew him from his frequent visits to the emergency room, where he would arrive almost unconscious, suffering from respiratory failure and with high levels of carbon dioxide in his blood. He was always treated in the same way: one of the interns would insert a rigid tube into Albie's windpipe through one of his nostrils, and allow him to spend the night sleeping at the hospital. The treatment always ended with Albie waking up alert and healthy the next morning, whereupon the tube would be removed from his throat. Every time Albie was admitted to the hospital, Read would gather all the new interns around his bed to show them the strange phenomenon, and conduct a heated debate on the possible physiological reasons for it.

Colin Sullivan was the engineer of the group, specializing in tubes, valves, and connectors, and Hensley was the "brains," spending more time in the library than in the laboratory. On one of Albie C.'s frequent visits, Hensley was just returning from the library with a copy of the *Bulletin de Physiopathologie Respiratoire* from 1972, which included the papers presented at the symposium organized by Lugaresi and his colleagues in Rimini. This was the same issue that had changed Eliot

Phillipson's medical career. Reading these papers shed new light on Albie C.'s illness. It was suddenly evident that Albie was not losing consciousness—he was suffering from sleep apnea syndrome. Because of this insight, in 1974, sleep recordings were carried out on a sleep apnea syndrome patient for the first time in Australia.

Albie C.'s sleep recordings led Read's group to change direction and deal intensively with the physiology of sleep in general, and respiratory function during sleep in particular. Encouraged by Read, who placed considerable importance on sleep apnea research, Sullivan completed his doctoral thesis and joined Eliot Phillipson's laboratory in Toronto. The three years Sullivan spent there yielded an abundance of findings and scientific papers, convincing him that his scientific future was permanently tied to sleep apnea syndrome.

Sullivan returned to Australia in 1978 and set up a sleep laboratory in an abandoned storeroom at the University of Sydney, where he continued to study respiratory control during sleep. He did not limit himself to research, however, and started looking for sleep apnea patients even before he had suitable equipment for sleep examinations. The first piece of equipment he used was a clumsy machine that had been constructed at Read's laboratory for making sleep recordings in infants. To conduct examinations on adult patients, Sullivan would borrow the university's truck, drive to the children's hospital five kilometers away, load the trolley with the recording machine onto the truck, and drive back to the adult hospital. There he would drag it along the corridors to the pulmonary function laboratory, where he used a crowded corner to conduct examinations on sleep apnea patients. These would begin at eight or nine o'clock in the evening and continue throughout the night. Some nights, Sullivan would go home for some rest and then return to the hospital in the early hours of the morning to dismantle the mobile laboratory before the pulmonary staff arrived. A single electric cable left lying around would be sufficient for the head of the pulmonary laboratory to explode in anger and threaten to put an immediate stop to Sullivan's nocturnal activities.

In spite of the underground conditions, by 1979 Sullivan had diagnosed eight patients with obstructive sleep apnea syndrome. Research conditions improved considerably in 1980 when the sleep laboratory was relocated to the university and situated near the animal research laboratory. Here Sullivan could study humans during the night and dogs and sheep during the day. The number of sleep examinations in sleep apnea patients gradually increased, while research activity into subjects related to respiratory and airway control during sleep continued. In March 1980, Sullivan organized the first international conference in Australia on respiratory function during sleep, which was attended by the top researchers worldwide.

Sullivan clearly remembers when he first came up with the notion that introducing pressurized airflow via the nostrils could prevent apneas during sleep. He was doodling a sketch of the upper airways on a sheet of paper, and in his mind's eye he tried to pinpoint the exact location where the obstruction occurs during sleep. In that instant, he formulated the idea that applying counterpressure on that point by introducing airflow would prevent the collapse. He kept the idea to himself and began investigating how to make a machine that would do such a thing. One of the first problems was constructing an airtight mask. One day, while visiting Read's laboratory, Sullivan noticed the lab technicians using liquid adhesive to seal a mask being placed on a sheep's snout. He tested the liquid adhesive on his face and, after ensuring that there were no side effects, started preparing a mask for respiration under pressure for a sleeping human. He used a vacuum cleaner motor with variable speeds to pump the air through a pipe. To the end of the pipe he attached soft plastic tubes for insertion into the patient's nostrils, and then connected another tube for exhaling. All that remained was to wait for a suitable opportunity to test the idea, and it was not long in coming.

In June 1981, Sullivan was asked to examine a construction worker who kept falling asleep on scaffolding. The man was forty-five years old, and although he was not overweight his sleep examination revealed that he suffered from severe sleep apnea syndrome. Sullivan recommended that he undergo a tracheostomy, but the man refused, so Sullivan decided to try treating him with airflow.

When the fateful evening arrived, the air compressor was placed next to the patient's bed, the mask and the plastic tubes were sealed all around with liquid adhesive, the lights were switched off, and everyone waited tensely for the experiment to begin. The man himself ignored the fuss being made over him and immediately fell asleep, as was his wont. Soon his snores could be heard from afar. After about ten minutes of prolonged apneas, Sullivan gradually increased the speed of the air compressor. The pressure rose slowly, and several minutes later, to everyone's astonishment, the man began breathing regularly. "The change was absolutely amazing," Sullivan recalls twenty-five years later. "Before we even had a chance to understand what had happened, the patient was already in REM sleep." The man breathed regularly and had no apneas at all. Undeniably, his breathing depended on the pressure of the air, because when it was reduced, the apneas reappeared, and when the pressure was increased once again, they disappeared.

The treatment was so remarkable that on that same night, even before the examination had ended, Sullivan retired to the next room and in the early hours of the morning finished drafting a paper on the treatment and its results, with recording machines creaking in the background as they documented one of the most important experiments ever conducted in any sleep laboratory.

When the man awoke in the morning, he was completely alert for the first time in several years, and he remained alert during the entire day. Sullivan initially thought to immediately publish the effect of treatment with CPAP as a one-case anecdote, which is fairly common in scientific publications. But after further thought he changed his mind, deciding to corroborate his finding with four additional patients. Sullivan professed that he examined the first three of these to convince himself of the validity of the findings, and the fourth to convince the editor of *The Lancet,* to whom he submitted his paper. Incidentally, one of the five patients was a thirteen-year-old boy who suffered from severe sleepiness and was considered retarded. Treatment with CPAP not only eliminated his sleepiness, it also removed the label of retardation that had been attached to him. One of the other patients was the famed Albie C.

The paper by Sullivan and his colleagues was published in *The Lancet* in 1981, and it became a milestone in the history of sleep apnea syndrome. Like Terry Young's article on the civil service workers in

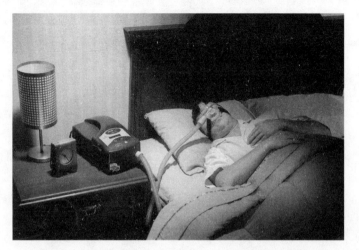

A patient being treated with CPAP to prevent sleep apnea

Wisconsin, Sullivan's paper has been quoted thousands of times, and it completely changed the approach to treatment of sleep apnea patients.

The Sleep of Mr. H.

Happily, the Technion Sleep Laboratory was one of the first in the world to learn the secret of Colin Sullivan's treatment. This was thanks to both the determination and the financial backing of one of our patients, Mr. H. He was one of the first to be diagnosed at our sleep laboratory with severe sleep apnea syndrome. Every night, Mr. H. had more than four hundred apneas during his sleep. As his sleep recording also showed a severe disorder of his heart rate, he underwent an immediate tracheostomy. But some years later, complications and infection made it necessary to close the stoma, which caused an immediate reappearance of the syndrome. Mr. H. then embarked upon a long series of surgical procedures on his upper airways, which did nothing to improve his condition. At one of our consultations I told him about the new Australian discovery, and without hesitation Mr. H. proposed that we contact Dr. Sullivan to inquire about the possibility of his coming to Israel with one of his

new respiration machines. Mr. H. offered to absorb all the expenses involved. It turned out that Sullivan's right-hand man, Ron Grunstein, had
relatives in Israel, and so it fortunately came to pass that he landed here
just two weeks after our telephone conversation, carrying a large metal
box containing the new wonder machine.

As we quickly discovered, the most complicated aspect of preparing the patient for respiratory treatment during sleep was fitting the mask
to the patient's face. A thick layer of a viscous rubberlike compound had
to be applied to his face and then allowed to dry. This formed a mask on
the patient's face that was then peeled off, and the air compressor tube
was attached to it. Mr. H. was a tower of strength, and his reward was not
long in coming. Once he had fallen asleep, Dr. Grunstein gradually increased the air pressure inside the mask until the apneas disappeared
completely, and the sleep recordings showed signs of turbulent REM
sleep. But unlike the first REM sleep of a normal night, which usually
lasts only a few minutes, Mr. H.'s REM sleep continued for almost one
and a half hours. I had never observed such prolonged REM sleep.
Grunstein was not surprised; he told us that one of the first observations
they had made of patients who had undergone this treatment was an immediate entry into a prolonged REM or deep sleep at the moment the
apneas disappeared. It is almost certain that this is an immediate compensation for a long period of the normal amount of REM and deep
sleep being prevented by the apneas. When he awoke, Mr. H. sponta-
neously exclaimed, "That was a dream of a sleep!" A few days later, Dr.
Grunstein returned to Australia, leaving the CPAP machine with Mr. H.

According to Sullivan himself, despite its remarkable success, he
did not imagine that CPAP would become the most widely used treatment for sleep disordered breathing. He feared that as soon as the problem of excessive daytime sleepiness was resolved, patients would find it
difficult to fall asleep wearing the mask. The first home CPAP machine
was manufactured in 1981 after a patient asked to continue treatment at
home. By 1985, only ten more patients were treated with positive air
pressure in their homes. But a couple of years later the first commercial
machines were developed for home use, and the treatment gained
tremendous success. Tens of thousands of machines are sold worldwide

every year nowadays, and there is no dispute that respiration with positive air pressure is the most effective treatment for sleep apnea.

Most patients use a CPAP machine nightly, taking it with them when they sleep away from home. Neither they nor their sleeping partners can any longer imagine life without regular airflow during their sleep.

Consenting to Treatment—A Subject Calling for Improvement

The efficacy of CPAP for treatment of sleep apnea has been proved in hundreds of studies and reports. The catch, however, is that many patients are not prepared to sleep every night wearing a mask with a tube dangling from it connected to an air compressor. At least half, in fact, of all sleep apnea patients who need treatment refuse CPAP, several studies show.

Sleep doctors tend to view the lack of enthusiasm among sleep apnea patients about the CPAP mask as an almost personal affront. Yet they should bear in mind that sleep apnea patients are not the only ones who don't always do what their doctors know is best for them. Fewer than half of all hypertension patients take their medication precisely as instructed by their doctors. In fact, patients who follow medical treatment instructions to the letter are the exception rather than the rule.

There are also particular aspects of CPAP treatment that limit patients' willingness to use the machine. The most important of these is how the machine is adapted to each patient, which is not at all simple. At our laboratory, when the decision is made to treat with CPAP, the patient is invited to spend another night at the sleep laboratory to determine the required treatment pressure. Most laboratories in the United States, however, to save the expense of an additional night at the sleep laboratory, diagnose the syndrome and adapt treatment pressure in the course of one night. In a "split night" of this kind, the patient sleeps for the first three hours of the examination with no treatment of any sort. If the doctors observe apneas of a severity greater than a specified limit, they rouse the patient, fit a mask to his or her face, and tell the poor person to go back to sleep for a further three hours so they can determine the treatment pressure. This does not exactly heighten the willingness of patients to receive the treatment.

Our experience shows that how willing patients are to accept treatment depends a great deal on how they feel after the first night of sleep wearing a CPAP mask. The greater the contrast between feeling fatigued and sleepy after a night with no treatment and feeling alert and energetic after treatment, the greater the likelihood that the patient will consent to sleep with a mask at home. Some patients awaken from their first night's sleep with CPAP with a sense that they have never slept so well. It is easy to convince these patients that the treatment is necessary. But if patients experience difficulty adjusting to the mask or the air pressure, or their sleep was too short, as is the case with split nights, their subjective feelings the next day are no different from how they feel after a night without treatment. Our experience is that 20 to 30 percent of all patients refuse treatment with CPAP immediately after the first night of adaptation. Patients who reject the treatment are impervious to the benefits they may derive from using what they view as the "bothersome" mask. And even initial consent to treatment does not guarantee that patients will continue with it. Up to half of all patients abandon the machine within the first few weeks.

This disturbing fact was unknown during the early years of the machine's use. At first, data on the extent of CPAP use came from personal reports by the patients. These reports, it turns out, were always exaggerated. Only when usage meters were installed in CPAP machines was it discovered that the actual usage was always lower than what patients reported. Some used the machine for only two or three hours a night, or for two to three nights a week, but they reported full and regular use every night.

Waking Up with a Smile

How can levels of consent to use CPAP be increased and how can the crisis of the first few weeks be overcome?

The attitudes of the medical and technical staff at the sleep laboratory and their involvement in the treatment procedure have a considerable influence. The procedure begins with an explanation that must be
provided simply and clearly to the patients and their sleeping partners
about the technical aspects of the treatment and its clinical importance.
The patient has to comprehend that the purpose of the treatment is
twofold: to improve sleep during the night and quality of life during the
day, and to prevent the negative effects of apneas, especially on the cardiovascular system.

Once the first obstacle has been surmounted and the patient has
consented to the first test to determine the treatment pressure, adaptation
has to be carried out meticulously, ensuring the patient's maximal comfort during sleep. This is where the sleep technician responsible for the
examination enters the picture. On the night of the adaptation, attention
to detail is essential, including properly fitting the mask and the straps
that secure it to the patient's face, muffling the noise of the air compressor, and accurately setting the treatment pressure. A patient, persuasive
technician is as critical to the success of the treatment as the doctor.

Determining the treatment pressure is not a simple matter and
must be done with care. As soon as apneas appear after the onset of
sleep, the pressure is gradually increased inside the CPAP mask, to the
point at which all the apneas disappear. Apneas tend to become more severe during REM sleep in overweight subjects, and when patients are
sleeping on their backs, so the technician has to meticulously monitor
sleep stages and positions throughout the night. If the apneas reappear,
the pressure has to be further increased until they disappear again.
Hence, any examination to determine treatment pressure must include
the REM sleep stage, and preferably also changes in sleeping positions.
At the end of the examination, the optimal treatment pressure is determined. If adaptation of treatment pressure is successful, the patient will
wake up smiling.

But the improvement is not always so dramatic or so immediate. In
such cases acclaim and enthusiasm are replaced by complaints that
"The mask was pressing on the bridge of my nose," or "I woke up several times because of dryness in my nose," or "The air was too cold," or

"It felt as though I was almost suffocating." Some patients even remove the mask in the middle of the night. All patients who find the experience difficult require close attendance and counseling for a few weeks to help them adjust to the machine and persevere with the treatment. A skilled technician can easily identify the causes of discomfort and considerably alleviate them. Pressure on the bridge of the nose can be reduced by changing mask size or type, or by loosening the straps; many patients are not even aware that there are several kinds of masks that come in different sizes. Dryness in the nose and feelings of coldness can be relieved by heating and moistening the air with a special attachment. Patients who find it difficult to adjust to the CPAP pressure and experience anxiety about suffocating can be helped if the pressure is reduced during the first nights and they are given a chance to adapt gradually to increasing pressures.

In particularly difficult cases, a "smart" CPAP machine can be used. With regular CPAP machines, treatment pressure is determined experimentally by gradually adjusting it and observing the effect on the apneas. From then on, the patient uses the same treatment pressure, whether sleeping on the back or the side, and whether he or she consumed any alcohol before going to sleep or not. A "smart" CPAP machine, in contrast, increases or reduces the pressure as required, using airflow sensors to make automatic adjustments. If the sensors identify apneas, an electronic command is relayed to the compressor to increase the pressure until the apneas completely disappear. If they identify a prolonged period with no apneas, the pressure inside the mask is reduced. In this way, treatment is adjusted according to variations in severity of the syndrome due to changes in body weight, position during sleep, or different sleep stages.

Whether the "smart" machines are more beneficial than the dumb ones appears to depend on the type of patient. No significant difference has been found in the efficacy of treatment, either in frequency of apneas and drops in blood oxygen saturation levels, or in the degree of improvement in daytime symptoms. Most comparisons have shown that the "smart" machines generally supply a lower pressure than the one determined on the night of adaptation. A reduced treatment pressure is a particular advantage to patients who experience feelings of suffocation and claustrophobia when using the machine, and those who have apneas especially when sleeping on their backs.

One of the questions sleep apnea patients ask most often about CPAP machines is what minimal time of use per night is required to improve sleep and daytime functioning. There is no conclusive answer to this question, but a significant correlation has been shown between duration of CPAP use and patients' quality of life and degree of daytime sleepiness. Hence, the longer the machine is used every night, the greater the probability of normal functioning during the day. Whether there is any association between the amount of CPAP use and the degree of cardiovascular disease has not yet been shown.

Diagnosis and Treatment Under One Roof

The motivation and skill of the technical staff at the sleep laboratory undoubtedly plays an important role in the success of treatment with CPAP. But the treatment is not always the responsibility of the sleep laboratory. In many places, especially in the United States, diagnosis of sleep apnea and treatment with CPAP are carried out by two different, independent bodies. Whereas diagnosis of the syndrome and determination of the treatment pressure are carried out at the sleep laboratory by sleep disorder specialists, the machine itself is provided to the patient by a different entity, completely separate from the sleep laboratory. This is usually a company that specializes in home treatments of various kinds, and one of its activities is the supply of CPAP machines. This situation has a significant impact on treatment compliance, as I discovered some years ago.

Following publication of my book *The Enchanted World of Sleep* in 1996, I was invited to Los Angeles to lecture on sleep apnea syndrome. Although my talk had not been specially advertised, the hall was, to my surprise, completely full. It was only after I had finished the lecture and was taking questions that I discovered why the event was so popular. Many of the attendees were sleep apnea patients who had come for an update on their illness, especially on its treatment. Although all had been diagnosed accurately and professionally at sleep laboratories and had been advised to use the CPAP machine, hardly any of them had actually used it. The reasons for this were eloquently expressed by a woman around sixty years old who, judging by her size and the fact that she spent most of the lecture in a deep sleep, presumably suffered from severe sleep apnea syndrome. She explained that when CPAP had been recommended to her, she had been referred to a home-equipment supplier to get her machine. Following a telephone conversation with the company, a large package containing the machine was delivered to her by courier. A technician from the company arrived at her home a week later, gave her a brief explanation of how to use the machine, adjusted it to the suitable pressure, and left. On the very first night she realized that there was air leakage from the mask, and wearing it did not help. Despite repeated calls to the company, her predicament was not addressed, and she did not use the machine again. In fact, she had come to my lecture to learn from me how the leakage could be overcome. She sounded surprised and even annoyed when I explained that there were several types of mask and that she could try a different one, more comfortable and more airtight than the one that had been supplied. Many other people asked for advice on a variety of problems they had encountered in using the CPAP machine. Clearly, they had no one to turn to for advice and assistance.

The attitude toward the patient is entirely different when both diagnosis and treatment are carried out under one roof. For companies specializing in the supply of home equipment, CPAP is just one of many home treatments, but for the specialists at the sleep laboratory, sleep apnea patients are foremost, because they are about 80 percent of all the patients examined there. Moreover, experience in treating a large number of patients with the same symptoms leads to increased professionalism and skill in solving problems that arise when using the machine. One of my friends, R.K. from Washington, had suffered from sleep apnea for several years and used a CPAP machine every night. One day he urgently called me because of an unexpected problem with it. As is our custom in such cases, I referred him to the person responsible for CPAP at the Technion Sleep Laboratory, who solved his problem almost immediately via e-mail. Impressed with the speed of service and good advice, R.K. called me and suggested that the Technion Sleep Laboratory establish a paid advice service for CPAP users in the United States. He was greatly surprised when I told him that we have indeed been involved in providing diagnosis and treatment services in the United States for about a year.

The Sleep HealthCenter—The American Effort

In the summer of 1996, I lectured in Boston before a large audience of Technion graduates and friends in my capacity as dean of the Faculty of Medicine. When I spoke about the Technion and its contribution to the state of Israel, I also described the activities of the Technion Sleep Medicine Center. Sleep always arouses great interest, and even those who had slept through most of my lecture suddenly woke up.

I related with some pride that the center at the Technion operates laboratories for diagnosis of sleep disorders in Haifa, Jerusalem, Holon, Tel Aviv, and Hadera. Many more people have been examined at these laboratories than in any other laboratory or center worldwide. I also expanded on my belief that sleep medicine cannot merely diagnose the disorder but must also complement the diagnosis with treatment.

At the end of the lecture a member of the audience approached me and introduced himself as David Barone, a Technion graduate, and asked me whether a similar service existed in the United States. When I told him that although there are about three thousand sleep laboratories in the country, they are relatively small and for the most part deal with diagnosis only, his response was to ask whether I personally had considered replicating the Technion model in the United States. I was sure he was joking, so I answered him jestingly that my business acumen is rather poor. But his question had been in earnest, and he added, "I will contribute to the business aspects." He was indeed absolutely serious. A week later he visited Israel for a crash course in sleep medicine and to closely observe our work methods, and within a few months sufficient funds had been raised to establish the Sleep HealthCenter in Boston. Happily, we were able to recruit David White of Harvard University, who agreed to accept the position of clinical director of the center.

The center's first laboratory was in Boston, co-founded with Brigham and Women's Hospital, and it was immediately followed by several other laboratories where thousands of people are diagnosed and treated every year. The center's slogan is: "Better sleep. Better health. It's that simple."

18

A Whole New Understanding

By any possible yardstick, the past ten to fifteen years have seen a complete turnabout in medicine's approach to sleep apnea syndrome. From being considered a rare and exotic condition it has become a routine term in the lexicons of physicians from many and varied branches of medicine. This change did not come about easily. Doctors are not readily impressed by new syndromes or treatments, and it takes a long time for scientific papers to change the characteristics of a diagnosis and treatment. It is therefore hardly surprising that seventeen years elapsed between the establishment in 1961 of the American Sleep Research Society—the sole function of which was research—and the founding of the American Sleep Disorders Association in 1978.

There is no doubt that Terry Young's 1993 article in the *New England Journal of Medicine* on the prevalence of sleep apnea syndrome, and the accompanying editorial by Eliot Phillipson asserting that it is a central public health problem, gave the syndrome an official imprimatur in the medical community. Since then the number of scientific articles on the syndrome has increased annually, as have the number of physicians dealing with it and the number of scientific journals concerned with sleep disorders in general. We can also learn something of this from the increasing number of physicians who each year participate in scientific conferences on the subject of sleep apnea syndrome and its consequences.

Today, these conferences are attended not by sleep experts only, but also by physicians from a multitude of disciplines.

Some years ago, when we examined which doctors referred patients suspected of having sleep apnea syndrome for examination at the Technion Sleep Laboratory, we found that the list was headed by ear, nose, and throat (ENT) specialists, because, among other things, they were the first to discover the economic potential of the snoring population. It was only later that doctors from other branches of medicine, like pulmonary specialists and, more recently, family doctors, woke up to this. The last to discover the syndrome and its effects were the cardiologists, even though epidemiological studies show that almost half the patients visiting cardiology clinics suffer from sleep disordered breathing; until recently, cardiologists remained indifferent to the syndrome.

Why is the cardiologists' position so important? First, their waiting rooms are populated by the greatest number of patients at high risk of sleep apnea syndrome. One needs only to circulate a short sleep questionnaire in cardiology wards to know that 40 to 50 percent of coronary heart disease patients are also afflicted with sleep apnea syndrome. Only a few of them are properly diagnosed today, and even fewer are given suitable treatment. Second, cardiologists are also the physicians who treat the syndrome's consequences, because sleep apnea patients reach them after they are affected by coronary heart disease or have their first heart attack. In these cases the syndrome is diagnosed too late, when the damage to the cardiovascular system has already been done.

The acceptance of sleep apnea syndrome by the medical community will be completed only when the first sleep laboratory is set up in a cardiology ward, and in my view that day is not far off.

CPAP: Is It Too Late?

We can assume from the accumulated knowledge on the syndrome and its clinical implications that damage to the cardiovascular system starts to accrue on the first night that the apneas appear. From then on, night after night, the blood vessels and the heart are exposed to the aggression of the free radicals that are formed with the ebb and flow of the patient's blood oxygen saturation level. People come for their first diagnosis only when the symptoms of snoring and daytime sleepiness start bothering them or their partners. This usually happens only many years after the patient has begun to have apneas during sleep.

A Swedish study found that people who snore loudly night after night, and who even reported fatigue and sleepiness, did not go for a sleep examination of their own accord. The average age of patients examined at sleep laboratories in different parts of the world is somewhere around fifty, so we can state with a high degree of certainty that people with sleep apnea syndrome experience sleep respiratory disorders for at least ten years before they are diagnosed and treated. It is entirely possible that the cumulative damage of those ten years, between the syndrome's first appearance and its diagnosis, is irreversible.

There are signs that the delay in treatment is significant in some patients at least, and evidence of this can be found in mortality studies. The average mortality age in sleep apnea patients is approximately sixty-five, regardless of whether they were treated with CPAP or not. Surprisingly, a French study that followed up treated sleep apnea patients showed that the average age of patients who died was younger, at 61.5 years, than that of our untreated patients. How can these findings be explained? It is quite possible that CPAP treatment, which came on the scene at least ten years after the appearance of the syndrome, does not arrest the damage to the cardiovascular system. Therefore, treatment of the syndrome should be begun at as young an age as possible. This should not be construed to mean that treating the syndrome at a later age is valueless. The disappearance of daytime sleepiness and fatigue and the enhancement of daytime functioning completely justify the inconvenience of wearing a CPAP mask while sleeping.

But in contrast to the immediate improvement in the patient's quality of life resulting from the treatment, we do not have an answer to the question of how efficacious CPAP is in reducing the cardiovascular risk, especially if we bear in mind that the majority of patients do not use the machine throughout the night, and not even every night. Jan Hedner and his group reported that CPAP can be perceived as only "half" a treatment of sleep apnea syndrome, as the patients are not actually being treated for half the time. Does this provide the patient with sufficient defense against the consequences of nightly hypoxia? We cannot say so with any certainty. The findings of the Wisconsin studies and the American Sleep Heart Health Study showed that even a small number of sleep apneas—ten to fifteen an hour—holds a significant risk of cardiovascular disease. What, then, is the significance of a treatment that reduces the number of apneas from sixty to twenty, or even ten, per hour?

In contrast, we cannot ignore the convincing proof that CPAP treatment reduced the blood pressure of sleep apnea patients and even prevented ischemic episodes in the sleep of heart patients who also suffered from sleep apnea syndrome. As I mentioned earlier, our studies have shown that CPAP reduced the "aggressiveness" of the white blood cells taking part in the sclerotic process and brought about an increased nitric oxide concentration in the patients' blood. It is therefore possible that the treatment reduces continued damage to the cardiovascular system, albeit without "healing" the damage already caused. We can assume that had CPAP treatment been commenced earlier, closer to the first appearance of the sleep breathing disorders, its efficacy would have been far greater.

Apneas and the Insurance Companies

In order to diagnose the syndrome as close as possible to the time of its appearance, a real revolution is needed in the approach to it on the part of doctors, health maintenance organizations, and insurance companies. Doctors must take a more active approach to diagnosing the syndrome. They must not wait until a patient or a spouse comes to them with a complaint; they must investigate their patients' sleeping habits, their snoring, the degree of their daytime fatigue, and so on. This active investigation is particularly important in populations defined by a high risk of sleep apnea syndrome, including overweight patients, people with airway blockages, the children of sleep apnea patients, and young people with hypertension or heart disease.

By the same token, no less important is the policy of the medical insurance companies. Most insurance companies do not have a planned policy of preventive medicine whose aim is the reduction of future risk of disease. In many cases the insurers have no desire to invest in tests that will prevent illness in another ten or fifteen years, for by then the policy holder may have moved to another insurance company. Several studies that have examined the health system's costs for sleep apnea syndrome patients before and after treatment showed that these are erroneous assumptions.

Meir Kryger of Winnipeg exploited the fact that records of all the health expenses for the citizens of Manitoba were computerized, and he examined the medical expenses of 344 sleep apnea syndrome patients for the year prior to diagnosis, and then compared them with the same expenses two years after the patients had begun CPAP treatment. He also compared patients' expenses before treatment with those of a control group that was randomly sampled from the general population. Medical expenses included payments for examinations, medication, visits to doctors, and hospitalizations. The findings were compelling. Prior to diagnosis, a person with sleep apnea syndrome cost the Manitoba health system $260 a year *more* than a person with the same body mass and of the same age who did not suffer from the syndrome. Two years after the commencement of CPAP treatment the difference was reduced to $174. When Kryger and his colleagues compared the medical expenses of patients who persevered with the treatment with those who stopped it, he found that the reduction in expenses applied only to the persevering patients.

Similar findings were reported in Israel by a group led by Asher Tal and Ariel Tarasiuk of Ben-Gurion University of the Negev, Beersheba. From health maintenance organization records, Tarasiuk, Tal, and their colleagues examined all the medical expenses of 237 children between the ages of one and eighteen who had been diagnosed with sleep apnea syndrome between the years 1998 and 2000 at the Soroka Medical Center in Beersheba. The expense records included the number of hospitalizations, the number of hospitalization days, visits to a pediatrician, and costs of medication. In comparison with the medical expenses of 1,149 children of the same age who were free of the syndrome, the expenses of those with the syndrome were 225 percent higher. One child out of every ten with sleep apnea syndrome was hospitalized at least once, in comparison with six out of one hundred children in the control group. The hospitalization duration of children with sleep apnea syndrome was longer as well: 0.23 days compared with 0.16 days for children from the control group. The syndrome sufferers also visited the hospital emergency room twice as often, and visited specialists almost four times as often, particularly visits to ENT specialists. In addition, they incurred higher expenses due to special tests and medication.

Early diagnosis of children with sleep apnea syndrome, therefore, is of great importance, not only because of the syndrome's effect on their health and scholastic achievement, but also because of their medical expenses.

If we take into account that diagnosis of the syndrome in adults is made, in most cases, only some ten to twenty years after the onset of respiratory disorders, then the health system spends vast sums on these patients before they are even diagnosed. To cut medical expenses, there should be no wait for the patient's complaints of snoring and sleepiness, and surveys should be initiated to diagnose sleep apnea syndrome in high-risk populations at as early an age as possible. Only thus can we make an early identification of those who, in the fullness of time, will become a burden upon the health system, and at the same time prevent future incidence of disease.

Apneas and Medical Education

Widening awareness of sleep apnea syndrome and its clinical implications mandates the subject's inclusion in the medical school syllabus. Today's medical students are given almost no training in the field of sleep and sleep disorders. The American Sleep Disorders Association has conducted three comprehensive surveys that examined the scope of teaching the subject of sleep in American medical schools. The first, in 1978, included 116 medical schools, and it found that in half of them the subject was not taught at all, while in one-third it was taught in the scope of one to four hours throughout all the years of study. Even when the subject was taught, it was done so incidentally as part of courses like physiology, pharmacology, or neural sciences, by teachers untrained in sleep medicine. Only in 10 percent of the medical schools was the study of sleep and its disorders given a passing grade. Not surprisingly, this 10 percent comprised schools in which there were active sleep researchers. A further survey, ten years later, included 126 medical schools, and its findings were almost identical to those of the previous one. According to the second survey, the number of schools that did not teach anything at all about sleep dropped to 37 percent, but the schools where the subject was taught were still content with less than two hours on it through all the years of study. A third survey showed that in 2000, too, no change in this state of affairs had taken place. Medical students who completed their studies at the end of the second millennium studied sleep and sleep disorders for only two hours. Other countries have reported similar findings. In Israeli medical schools, too, with the exception of the Technion and Ben-Gurion University, the field is almost not taught at all.

What is the reason for the tremendous gap between the scientific progress made in sleep research and disorders and the absence of recognition of the subject's importance in the medical schools? As a former dean of the Technion Faculty of Medicine, I feel that the reason is not the attitude of medical educators toward sleep medicine, but rather the slowness and conservatism that characterize medical teaching programs in general. The field of medical education has been defined by one expert as "a confederation of semi-autonomous dukedoms in which the dukes (the medical school department heads) bypass the princes (the deans) and the kings and queens (the university presidents) who they are supposed to obey."

What this expert meant was that the traditional medical school departments, such as physiology, anatomy, pharmacology, and clinical departments like internal medicine, neurology, or psychiatry, are in constant competition over budgets, posts, fields of research, and even teaching hours. As a result, no department is prepared to give up teaching hours for the benefit of another department or for the benefit of a

new subject of study, lest they be deducted from its own posts or budgets, and consequently diminish its standing in the school. Thus any
change in the medical school syllabus is bound up in a struggle of titans
in which the dean of the faculty, or the dean's deputy for teaching, plays
a decisive role.

In order to diagnose the syndrome as early as possible, the family
doctor needs a far greater awareness of sleep disorders and the importance of healthy sleep for human functioning. We have seen this every
now and then when we opened a new laboratory for the diagnosis of
sleep disorders in Israel. In the early years of the Technion Sleep Laboratory in Haifa, when it was the only one in Israel, one could obtain the
distinct impression that only the residents of Haifa and its environs suffered from sleep apnea syndrome or other sleep disorders. The reason
for this was that patients from other parts of Israel did not come to us.
When the Tel Aviv branch of the laboratory was opened in 1985, it became clear, either to our relief or to our disappointment, that Tel Avivi-
ans suffer from sleep apnea syndrome to the same extent as the residents
of Haifa and the north of Israel. The same thing happened in Jerusalem
when we opened a laboratory there in 1990.

Others had similar experiences, the most notable of which was a
project called Walla Walla, after the township in a valley of the same
name in the southeastern corner of Washington State, in western America. Walla Walla, as its Native American name suggests, is located in a fertile valley abounding with water and thick vegetation, and whose source
of pride is the extensive cultural and artistic activity of its thirty thousand
inhabitants. Another source of the citizens' pride is the township's son,
Bill Dement, who followed his guide and mentor, Nathaniel Kleitman, as
the high priest of sleep research in the United States.

During one of his visits with his mother, Dement realized that in
his hometown there was no awareness of sleep disorders. In an examination he conducted in the town's biggest clinic, he found that only 2 out
of 725 patients who had visited the clinic over a year had been diagnosed
with sleep apnea syndrome. It was clear to Dement that Walla Walla's
family doctors were unaware of the problem. As the flag bearer of sleep
medicine in the United States, Dement set himself a special challenge: to

educate the inhabitants and doctors of his hometown to recognize the importance of sleep. Over a period of two years Dement and his team from the Stanford Sleep Disorders and Research Center instructed Walla Walla's family doctors in all matters pertaining to sleep and its disorders, and provided them with equipment for diagnosis. At the end of the two years it became clear that the peaceful citizens of Walla Walla had sleep apnea syndrome just like their fellows in other American towns and cities. By a relative estimate, the number of people referred for sleep examination in Walla Walla increased eightfold. Over the two-year period 350 sleep examinations were conducted, in which 293 patients were diagnosed with the syndrome. By the end of June 2001, 4,800 sleep examinations had been conducted in Walla Walla, revealing sleep apnea syndrome in 70 percent of the cases—and this in a town where only a few years earlier there had been only two cases.

There is a great disproportion between the size of the population suffering from sleep apnea syndrome and the number of doctors engaged in sleep medicine. Assuming that the incidence of the syndrome is only 4 percent of the adult population, then every member of the twenty-person team engaged in sleep medicine in Israel provides consultation, diagnosis, and treatment to thousands of sleep apnea patients. There is an urgent need to expand the circle of physicians engaged in providing initial advice on sleep disorders. Our own experience, and that of Walla Walla, shows that the person most suitable to act as the agent of sleep medicine is the family doctor or general practitioner, who knows his or her patients better than anyone else does. These relationships are intimate enough that the family doctor can frankly discuss with patients their nocturnal snoring, daytime sleepiness, and how much they enjoy their sex life. The family doctor is also able to undertake long-term follow-up of changes in patients' health and habits.

But of course turning the family doctor into an agent of sleep medicine calls for suitable training. Doctors' awareness of the syndrome must be heightened, and they must develop an ability to recognize people who are at high risk. The initial diagnosis can be made through structured clinical interviews or by using instruments for monitoring sleep breathing in the patient's home. The latent snorers who pass the first test

with the family doctor will be referred for further investigation and treatment with sleep specialists equipped with laboratories and sophisticated instruments. I do not reject the possibility that after acquiring skill
and experience in diagnosing sleep disorders, some family doctors will
be able to treat their own patients and follow them up over time. But following up sleep apnea syndrome patients, as it is practiced in general
today, calls for a change of attitude.

The Need for Medical Follow-up

Follow-up with patients, whether they have been treated or not, almost
goes without saying in medicine. Patients who have been diagnosed with
diabetes, hypertension, or depression are not left to fend for themselves
once their condition has been diagnosed and treatment prescribed for it.
The doctor's role does not end with signing the prescription for medication. Sadly, the situation is different for the majority of sleep apnea
syndrome patients. In sleep laboratories all over the world the sleep specialist's job is over the moment the sleep recording has been deciphered
and the diagnosis made. As we have seen, CPAP treatment is provided
outside the sleep laboratory by people who are not specialists in sleep
medicine and sleep disorders. In the best case, patients are given appropriate treatment, and in the worst are not treated at all, but in either event
they are not usually invited back for a follow-up examination, another interview, or even a courtesy visit to the sleep clinic to find out what has become of them.

   This custom exacts a high price from both patient and sleep specialist. The patient has no one to turn to for consultation, and there are
some who remain with this threatening machine in their home, in some
cases still in its original packing. The sleep specialist pays a no less significant price: it is hard to imagine scientific progress in any field of medicine without the ability to undertake a precise and accurate follow-up of
patients. In the present situation, the sleep specialist has a single photo-
copy of the patient's sleep situation, and on the basis of this tries to conclude how the sleep disorder began ten years earlier, and what may hap-

pen ten, twenty, or even thirty years in the future. A continuous flow of information is likely to enable the specialist to draw conclusions on any change in the severity of the syndrome and the degree of risk to the patient. It is small wonder that in studies on sleep disorders in the elderly, very few conclusions have been drawn on the significance of sleep disordered breathing in old age. The researchers simply did not have any information on the sleep functioning of those elderly people in their youth or in middle age.

Long-term studies in medicine are of decisive importance in identifying disease risk factors and in understanding their development processes. The most well-known example of this is the Framingham Heart Study. In 1948, the American Cardiac Institute embarked on an unparalleled project to identify the causes of cardiovascular disease, the incidence of which in the United States had constantly increased since the beginning of the twentieth century. To this end, the researchers recruited 5,209 healthy men and women between the ages of thirty and sixty-two from Framingham, Massachusetts. The survey population underwent clinical interviews and exacting medical examinations. From the study's inception, the subjects were examined and interviewed every two years, and in 1971 the second generation of Framingham subjects was recruited—5,124 children of participants in the first group. In the fifty years since the Framingham Heart Study got under way, it has yielded more than a thousand scientific papers in leading medical journals, and these have changed the face of medicine in the field of cardiovascular disease. The exacting examinations undergone by the Framingham subjects led to the identification of the main risk factors for cardiovascular disease, such as high blood pressure, high cholesterol levels, smoking, obesity, diabetes, and lack of physical exercise.

It is almost certain that if we were able to turn back the clock and start the Framingham Heart Study over, then in light of what we now know about the connection between sleep apnea and cardiovascular disease, every couple of years all its participants would spend a night or two at a sleep laboratory. But we can find some comfort in the fact that a somewhat late recognition of the importance of sleep has made some of the Framingham study subjects participants in the American Sleep

Heart Health Study that began in 1996. Sleep researchers from all over the world are eagerly awaiting the study's results.

What Does the Future Hold?

Great efforts are being made in laboratories the world over to solve the riddle of sleep apnea. Numerous researchers are making progress on the way the nerve fibers control the pharyngeal muscles, and in their opinion the secret of pharyngeal collapse is to be found in understanding the neural transmission that causes the muscles to relax. Others are making advances in the development of innovative methods for respiration during sleep that will make it easier for patients to get used to wearing the CPAP mask. And other researchers are investigating the interpersonal differences likely to teach us which patients will adapt to the syndrome without any other significant illness, and which ones are likely to suffer heart attacks or strokes at an early age. Probably within only a few years we will be able, with the help of a simple blood test, to tell a patient to what degree he or she is at cardiovascular risk from nightly apneas.

Diagnosing the syndrome, too, is undergoing a developmental upsurge. The vast number of patients still waiting for a diagnosis mandates a different approach to the diagnostic process. Reliable, inexpensive methods are needed to enable the family doctor and the general practitioner to determine, with a high degree of certainty, which patients should be referred for further investigation and treatment. There is also a need for enhancing and simplifying home testing methods to reduce their cost and help make them available to all. As a result of the tremendous effort being invested in the field, in just the past few years some eighty new patents related to diagnosing or treating sleep apnea syndrome have been registered annually. Our own laboratory has also joined the effort to develop accessible and inexpensive diagnostic tools with the aim of identifying large groups of people at high risk of the syndrome.

So far we have developed two innovative technologies. The SLP Company, a subsidiary of the Haifa Technion Sleep Laboratory, has developed a disposable measuring instrument called SleepStrip, known as the "electronic mustache" because of its appearance, that traces nasal airflow to keep track of full or partial apneas for the purpose of identifying people at high risk of sleep apnea syndrome. Another company, Itamar Medical Ltd., has built an instrument for diagnosing sleep apnea syndrome using technology developed at the Technion Sleep Laboratory for measuring peripheral arterial tone. Based on accurate measurement of changes in the diameter of arterioles in a finger, this technology enables tracing of even the slightest sleep apneas by identifying the awakenings at their conclusion. This identification is made possible by the activation of the autonomic nervous system upon awakening, which causes massive contraction of the peripheral blood vessels. The great advantage of this instrument, known as PAT (peripheral arterial tone), is the possibility of using recordings made from two fingers only, so that the patient can use the device without any technical assistance.

The growing use of devices like these will be a great help in the early identification of many sleep apnea patients, enabling doctors to follow them up at a very low cost. Medical and scientific attitudes toward sleep disorders have come a long way since the first theories on sleep respiratory disorders in Pickwickian patients. From an exotic condition that was thought to afflict only obese people, sleep apnea syndrome has become the driving force of sleep medicine. There are encouraging signs that sleep medicine will soon become a legitimate part of the medical profession. Every year for the past ten years there have been questions on sleep medicine in the U.S. National Medical Board exam. This forces medical students to pay much more attention to sleep and its disorders. Furthermore, President Bill Clinton, following the recommendation of a national congressional commission chaired by William Dement, signed a decree establishing a center for sleep research at the National Heart, Lung, and Blood Institute of the National Institutes of Health in 1993. One of the first decisions of this center was to facilitate the development of sleep medicine education in American medical schools. A recent study based on the U.S. National Ambulatory Medical Care Survey revealed that there had been a twelvefold increase in the reporting of sleep apnea cases between 1990 and 1998, from 110,000 patients to 1.3 million.

We have no definitive explanation of why humans' airways tend to collapse during sleep, but it almost certainly has something to do with our unique anatomy. In other animals, the hyoid bone—which provides support to the tongue—is firmly anchored to the skull and neck bones, but in humans it floats between soft flexible tissues. This special structure, which enables us to produce a wide range of sounds during the day, tends to contort and collapse during the night. It is therefore possible that sleep respiratory disorders are the price humans pay for their ability to talk. The voluntary respiratory centers located in the anterior lobe of the brain—the most recent in the brain's evolutionary development—are what enable us to simultaneously talk and breathe. The autonomic respiratory centers in the brain stem are far more rigid, and any slight disruption of the information reaching them from the innumerable sensors tracing respiratory movements, airflow, blood gas levels, or air pressure is liable to put them out of kilter. A better understanding of these mechanisms—the goal of the tremendous efforts being invested in scores of laboratories all over the world—will teach us much about how the brain copes with respiratory control during sleep. This, in turn, may one day allow us to completely prevent the nocturnal collapse of the airways, or at least reduce it to a minimum, and with it the many costly, life-threatening effects of the nightly struggle of so many patients with sleep apnea syndrome.

References

1. The Breath of Life

Foster, M. *Lectures on the History of Physiology in the Sixteenth and Eighteenth Centuries.* Cambridge, Cambridge University Press, 1901.

Fulton, J. F., and L. G. Wilson, eds. *Selected Readings in the History of Physiology,* 2d ed. Springfield, Ill., Charles C. Thomas, 1966.

Holmes, F. L. *Lavoisier and the Chemistry of Life.* Madison, University of Wisconsin Press, 1985.

2. Respiratory Control

Bulow, K., and D. H. Ingvar. "Respiration and state of wakefulness in normals, studied by spirography, capnography, and EEG: A preliminary report." *Acta Physiologica Scandinavica* 51 (1961): 230–38.

Cheyne, J. "A case of apoplexy in which the fleshy part of the heart was converted into fat." *Dublin Hospital Report* 2 (1818): 216–23.

Comroe, J. H., Jr. "Frankenstein, Pickwick, and Ondine's curse." *American Review of Respiratory Diseases* 111 (1975): 689–92.

Proctor, D. F., ed. *A History of Breathing Physiology.* New York, Marcel Dekker, 1995.

Reed, C. I., and N. Kleitman. "The effect of sleep on respiration." *American Journal of Physiology* 75 (1926): 600–608.

Sternbach, G. L., J. Cheyne, and W. Stokes. "Periodic respiration." *Journal of Emergency Medicine* 3 (1985): 233–36.

Stokes, W. *The Diseases of the Heart and Aorta.* Hodges & Smith, Dublin, Ireland, 1854.

Sugar, O. "In search of Ondine's curse." *Journal of the American Medical Association* 240 (1978): 236–37.

Ward, M. "Periodic respiration: A short historical note." *Annals of the Royal College of Surgeons of England* 52 (1973): 330–34.

Wells, H. H., J. Kattwinkel, and J. D. Morrow. "Control of ventilation of Ondine's curse." *Journal of Pediatrics* 96 (1980): 865–67.

241

3. The First Pickwickian

Catlin, G. *The Breath of Life.* New York, Wiley, 1861.

Dourmashkin, R. R. "What caused the 1918–30 epidemic of encephalitis lethargica?" *Journal of the Royal Society of Medicine* 90 (1997): 515–20.

Lavie, P. "Nothing new under the moon, historical accounts of sleep apnea syndrome." *Archives of Internal Medicine* 144 (1984): 2025–28.

Lavie, P. "The touch of Morpheus: Pre-twentieth century accounts of sleepy patients." *Neurology* 41 (1991): 1841–44.

Wells, W. A. "Some nervous and mental manifestations occurring in connection with nasal disease." *American Journal of Medical Sciences* (1898): 677–92.

4. Rediscovery of the Pickwickian Patient

Burwell, C., et al. "Extreme obesity associated with alveolar hypoventilation—a pickwickian syndrome." *American Journal of Medicine* 21 (1956): 811–18.

Drachman, D. B., and R. J. Gumnit. "Periodic alteration of consciousness in the 'pickwickian' syndrome." *Archives of Neurology* 6 (1962): 63–69.

Gastaut, H., C. A. Tassinari, and B. Duron. "Polygraphic study of the episodic diurnal and nocturnal (hypnic and respiratory) manifestations of the pickwick syndrome." *Brain Research* 1 (1966): 167–86.

Gerardy, W., D. Herberg, and H. M. Kuhn. "Vergleichende Untersuchungen der Lungenfunktion und des Elektroencephalogramms bei zwei Patienten mit pickwickian-Syndrom." *Zeitschrift fur klinische Medizin* 156 (1960): 362–80.

Hishikawa, Y., E. Furuya, and H. Wakamatsu. "Hypersomnia and periodic respiration—presentation of two cases and comment on the physio-pathogenesis of the pickwickian syndrome." *Folia Psychiatrica et Neurologica Japonica* 24 (1970): 163–73.

Jung, R., and W. Kuhlo. "Neurophysiological studies of abnormal night sleep and the pickwickian syndrome." In *Progress in Brain Research: Sleep Mechanisms,* vol. 18, ed. K. Akert, C. Bally, and J. P. Schade. Amsterdam, Elsevier, 1965, 140–59.

Lugaresi E., et al. "Effect of tracheostomy in hypersomnia with periodic respiration." *Electroencephalography & Clinical Neurophysiology* 30 (1971): 373–74.

Lugaresi E., et al., "Hypersomnia with periodic breathing: Periodic apneas and alveolar hypoventilation during sleep." *Bulletin of Physiopathologic Respiration* (Bulletin de Physiopathologie Respiratoire) 8 (1972): 1103–13.

5. Western Innovations

Dement, W. C. *Some Must Watch While Some Must Sleep*. San Francisco, Norton, 1974.

Guilleminault, C., and W. C. Dement, eds. *Sleep Apnea Syndromes*. New York, Alan R. Liss, 1978.

Guilleminault, C., F. Eldridge, and W. C. Dement. "Insomnia, narcolepsy, and sleep apneas." *Bulletin of Physiopathologic Respiration* (Bulletin de Physiopathologie Respiratoire) 8 (1972): 1127–38.

Guilleminault, C., F. L. Eldridge, and W. C. Dement. "Insomnia with sleep apnea: A new syndrome." *Science* 181 (1973): 856–58.

Kryger, M., et al. "Diagnosis of obstruction of the upper and central airways." *American Journal of Medicine* 61 (1976): 85–93.

Kryger, M., et al. "The sleep deprivation syndrome of the obese patients: A problem of periodic nocturnal upper airway obstruction." *American Journal of Medicine* 56 (1974): 531–39.

Orr, W. C., et al. "Hypersomnolent and nonhypersomnolent patients with upper airway obstruction during sleep." *Chest* 75 (1979): 418–22.

6. The Dog Dropped Off and the Experiment Woke Up

Elliott, A. R., et al. "Microgravity reduces sleep-disordered breathing in humans." *American Journal of Respiratory and Critical Care Medicine* 164 (2001): 478–85.

Guilleminault, C., et al. "A cause of excessive daytime sleepiness, the upper airway resistance syndrome." *Chest* 104 (1993): 781–87.

Lugaresi, E., et al. "Staging of heavy snorers' disease, a proposal." *Bulletin of European Physiopathology of Respiration* 19 (1983): 590–94.

Phillipson, E. A. "Control of breathing in sleep." *American Review of Respiratory Disease* 118 (1978): 909–39.

Phillipson, E. A., et al. "Ventilatory and waking responses to hypoxia in sleeping dogs." *Journal of Applied Physiology* 44 (1978): 512–20.

Phillipson, E. A., E. Murphy, and L. F. Kozar. "Regulation of respiration in sleeping dogs." *Journal of Applied Physiology* 40 (1976): 688–93.

Weitzman, E. D., et al. "The hypersomnia sleep-apnea syndrome: Site and mechanism of upper airway obstruction." *Transactions of the American Neurological Association* 102 (1977): 150–53.

White, D. P., et al. "Pharyngeal resistance in normal humans: Influence of gender, age, and obesity." *Journal of Applied Physiology* 58 (1985): 365–71.

7. From an Exotic Syndrome to a Public Health Issue

Guilleminault, C., and E. Lugaresi, eds. *Sleep-Wake Disorders, Natural History, Epidemiology, and Long-Term Evolution.* New York, Raven Press, 1983.

Kripke, D. F., et al. "Prevalence of sleep-disordered breathing in ages 40–64 years, a population-based survey." *Sleep* 20 (1997): 65–76.

Lavie, P. "Incidence of sleep apnea in a presumably healthy working population, a significant relationship with excessive daytime sleepiness." *Sleep* 6 (1983): 312–18.

Lindberg, E., and T. Gislason. "Epidemiology of sleep related obstructive breathing." *Sleep Medicine Reviews* 4 (2000): 411–33.

Partinen, M., et al. "Genetic and environmental determination of human sleep." *Sleep* 6 (1983): 179–85.

Young, T., et al. "The occurrence of sleep-disordered breathing among middle-aged adults." *New England Journal of Medicine* 328 (1993): 1230–35.

Young, T. B. "Epidemiology of sleep apnea, analytic epidemiology studies of sleep disordered breathing—what explains the gender difference in sleep disordered breathing?" *Sleep* 26 (1993): S1–2.

8. Risk Factors for Sleep Apnea

Baldwin, D. R., et al. "Comparative clinical and physiological features of Maori, Pacific Islanders, and Europeans with sleep related breathing disorders." *Respirology* 3 (1998): 253–60.

Gleeson, K., et al. "Breathing route during sleep." *American Review of Respiratory Diseases* 134 (1986): 115–20.

Hanly, P. J., and A. Pierratos. "Improvement of sleep apnea in patients with chronic renal failure who undergo nocturnal hemodialysis." *New England Journal of Medicine* 344 (2001): 102–7.

Metes, A., et al. "Snoring, apnea, and nasal resistance in men and women." *Journal of Otolaryngology* 20 (1991): 57–61.

Millman, R. P., et al. "Central sleep apnea in hypothyroidism." *American Review of Respiratory Diseases* 127 (1983): 504–7.

Mokdad, A. H., et al. "The spread of the obesity epidemic in the United States, 1991–1998." *Journal of the American Medical Association* 282 (1999): 1519–22.

Mortimore, I. L., et al. "Neck and total body fat deposition in nonobese and obese patients with sleep apnea compared with that in control subjects." *American Journal of Respiratory and Critical Care Medicine* 157 (1998): 280–83.

Olsen, K. D., E. B. Kern, and P. R. Westbrook. "Sleep and breathing distur-
bance secondary to nasal obstruction." *Otolaryngology, Head, and Neck
Surgery* 89 (1981): 804–10.

Pelttari, L., et al. "Upper airway obstruction in hypothyroidism." *Journal of
Internal Medicine* 236 (1994): 177–81.

Pillar, G., and P. Lavie. "Assessment of the role of inheritance in sleep apnea
syndrome." *American Journal of Respiratory and Critical Care Medicine*
151 (1995): 688–91.

Popovic, R. M., and D. P. White. "Influence of gender on waking genioglossal
electromyogram and upper airway resistance." *American Journal of Respiration and Critical Care Medicine* 152 (1995): 725–31.

Redline, S., and P. V. Tishler. "The genetics of sleep apnea." *Sleep Medicine Reviews* 4 (2000): 583–602.

Redline, S., et al. "Racial differences in sleep-disordered breathing in African-
Americans and Caucasians." *American Journal of Respiratory and Critical Care Medicine* 155 (1997): 186–92.

Scrima, L., P. G. Hartman, and F. C. Hiller. "Effect of three alcohol doses on
breathing during sleep in 30–49 year-old nonobese snorers and non-
snorers." *Alcohol Clinical and Experimental Research* 13 (1989): 420–27.

Weiss, V., et al. "Prevalence of the sleep apnea syndrome in acromegaly population." *Journal of Endocrinological Investigation* 23 (2000): 515–19.

Young, T., L. Finn, and H. Kim. "Nasal obstruction as a risk factor for sleep-
disordered breathing." *Journal of Allergy and Clinical Immunology* 99
(1997): S757–62.

9. The Syndrome's Symptoms

Dalmasso, F., and R. Prota. "Snoring: Analysis, measurement, clinical implications, and applications." *European Respiratory Journal* 9 (1996): 146–59.

Decary, A., I. Rouleau, and J. Montplaisir. "Cognitive deficits associated with
sleep apnea syndrome, a proposed neuropsychological test battery."
Sleep 23 (2000): 369–81.

Engleman, H. M., et al. "Cognitive function in the sleep apnea/hypopnea syndrome (SAHS)." *Sleep* 23 (2000): S102–8.

Ferini-Strambi, L., et al. "Snoring in twins." *Respiratory Medicine* 89 (1995):
227–40.

Guilleminault, C., et al. "Determinants of daytime sleepiness in obstructive
sleep apnea." *Chest* 94 (1988): 32–37.

Kim, H. C., et al. "Sleep-disordered breathing and neuropsychological deficits, a population-based study." *American Journal of Respiratory and Critical Care Medicine* 156 (1997): 1813–19.

Roehrs, T., et al. "Predictors of objective level of daytime sleepiness in patients with sleep-related breathing disorders." *Chest* 95 (1989): 1202–6.

10. The Price of Awakenings

Barbe, P. J., et al. "Automobile accidents in patients with sleep apnea syndrome, an epidemiological and mechanistic study." *American Journal of Respiratory and Critical Care Medicine* 158 (1998): 18–22.

Benbadis, S. R., et al. "Prevalence of daytime sleepiness in a population of drivers." *Neurology* 52 (1999): 209–10.

Fischer, J., and F. Raschke. "Economic and medical significance of sleep-related breathing disorders." *Respiration* 64 (1997): 39–44.

Luboshitzky, R., et al. "Decreased pituitary-gonadal secretion in men with obstructive sleep apnea." *Journal of Clinical and Endocrinological Metabolism* 87 (2002): 3394–98.

Ronald, J., et al. "Health care utilization in the 10 years prior to diagnosis in obstructive sleep apnea syndrome patients." *Sleep* 22 (1999): 225–29.

Stoohs, R. A., et al. "Sleep and sleep-disordered breathing in commercial long-haul truck drivers." *Chest* 107 (1995): 1275–82.

Teran-Santos, J., A. Jimenez-Gomez, and J. Cordero-Guevara. "The association between sleep apnea and the risk of traffic accidents." *New England Journal of Medicine* 340 (1999): 847–51.

Yang, E. H., et al. "Sleep apnea and quality of life." *Sleep* 23 (2000): 535–41.

11. At the Temple of Morpheus

Chervin, R. D. "Periodic leg movements and sleepiness in patients evaluated for Sleep-Disordered Breathing." *American Journal of Respiratory and Critical Care Medicine* 164 (2001): 1454–58.

Coren, S. *Sleep Thieves.* New York, Free Press, 1996.

Dement, W. C., and C. Vaughan. *The Promise of Sleep.* New York, Delacorte Press, 1999.

Gadoth, N., et al. "Clinical and polysomnographic characteristics of 34 patients with Kleine-Levin syndrome." *Journal of Sleep Research* 10 (2001): 337–41.

Peyron, C., et al. "A mutation in a case of early onset narcolepsy and a general-ized absence of hypocretin peptides in human narcoleptic brains." *Nature Medicine* 6 (2000): 991–97.

Thannickal, T. C., et al. "Reduced number of hypocretin neurons in human narcolepsy." *Neuron* 27 (2000): 469–74.

12. Children and Sleep Apnea

Acres, J. C., et al. "Breathing during sleep in parents of sudden infant death syn-drome victims." *American Review of Respiratory Diseases* 125 (1982): 163–66.

Chervin, R. D., et al. "Symptoms of sleep disorders, inattention, and hyper-activity in children." *Sleep* 20 (1997): 1185–92.

Eliaschar, I., et al. "Sleep apneic episodes as indications for adenotonsillec-tomy." *Acta Otolaryngol* 106 (1980): 492–96.

Gaultier, C. "Sleep apnea in infants." *Sleep Medicine Reviews* 3 (1999): 303–12.

Goh, D. Y. T., P. Galster, and C. L. Marcus. "Sleep architecture and respiratory disturbances in children with obstructive sleep apnea." *American Jour-nal of Respiratory and Critical Care Medicine* 162 (2000): 682–86.

Gozal, D. "Sleep-disordered breathing and school performance in children." *Pediatrics* 102 (1998): 616–20.

Gozal, D., and D. W. Pope, Jr. "Snoring during early childhood and academic performance at ages thirteen to fourteen years." *Pediatrics* 107 (2001): 1394–99.

Guilleminault, C., et al. "Apneas during sleep in infants, possible relationship with sudden infant death syndrome." *Science* 190 (1975): 677–79.

Guilleminault, C., R. Korobkin, and R. Winkle. "A review of 50 children with obstructive sleep apnea syndrome." *Lung* 159 (1981): 275–87.

Gunn, A., T. R. Gunn, and E. A. Mitchell. "Is changing the sleep environment enough? Current recommendations for SIDS." *Sleep Medicine Reviews* 4 (2000): 453–69.

Harper, R. M., et al. "Periodicity of sleep states is altered in infants at risk for the sudden infant death syndrome." *Science* 213 (1981): 1030–32.

Hoppenbrouwers, T., et al. "Sudden infant death syndrome: Sleep apnea and respiration in subsequent siblings." *Pediatrics* 66 (1980): 205–14.

Kahn, A., et al. "Polysomnographic studies of infants who subsequently died of sudden infant death syndrome." *Pediatrics* 82 (1988): 721–27.

Marcus, C. L. "Sleep-disordered breathing in children." *Current Opinions in Pediatrics* 12 (2000): 208–12.

Pinholster, G. "Multiple 'SIDS' case ruled murder." *Science* 268 (1995): 494.

Ramanathan, R., et al. "Cardiorespiratory events recorded on home monitors, comparison of healthy infants with those at increased risk for SIDS." *Journal of the American Medical Association* 285 (2001): 2199–2207.

Redline, S., et al. "Risk factors for sleep-disordered breathing in children, associations with obesity, race, and respiratory problems." *American Journal of Respiratory and Critical Care Medicine* 159 (1999): 1527–32.

Schechtman, V. L., et al. "Dynamics of respiratory patterning in normal infants and infants who subsequently died of the sudden infant death syndrome." *Pediatric Research* 40 (1996): 571–77.

Strohl, K. P., et al. "Obstructive sleep apnea in family members." *New England Journal of Medicine* 199 (1978): 969–73.

13. Sleep Apnea, the Heart, and the Blood Vessels

Bixler, E. O., et al. "Association of hypertension and sleep-disordered breathing." *Archives of Internal Medicine* 160 (2000): 2289–95.

Brooks, D., et al. "Obstructive sleep apnea as a cause of systemic hypertension: Evidence from a canine model." *Journal of Clinical Investigation* 99 (1997): 106–9.

Carlson, J. T., et al. "High prevalence of hypertension in sleep apnea patients independent of obesity." *American Journal of Respiratory and Critical Care Medicine* 150 (1994): 72–77.

Hla, K. M., et al. "Sleep apnea and hypertension, a population-based study." *Annals of Internal Medicine* 120 (1994): 382–88.

Lavie, P., and V. Hoffstein. "Sleep apnea syndrome: A possible contributing factor to resistant hypertension." *Sleep* 24 (2001): 721–25.

Mooe, T., et al. "Sleep-disordered breathing in men with coronary artery disease." *Chest* 10 (1996): 659–63.

Peled, N., et al. "Nocturnal ischemic events in patients with obstructive sleep apnea syndrome and ischemic heart disease, effects of continuous positive air pressure treatment." *Journal of the American College of Cardiology* 34 (1999): 1744–49.

Peppard, P. E., et al. "Longitudinal study of moderate weight change and sleep-disordered breathing." *Journal of the American Medical Association* 284 (2000): 3015–21.

Peppard, P. E., et al. "Prospective study of the association between sleep-disordered breathing and hypertension." *New England Journal of Medicine* 342 (2000): 1378–84.

Shahar, E., et al. "Sleep-disordered breathing and cardiovascular disease: Cross-sectional results of the Sleep Heart Health Study." *American Journal of Respiratory and Critical Care Medicine* 163 (2001): 19–25.

Phillips, R. A., et al. "The association of blunted nocturnal blood pressure dip and stroke in a multiethnic population." *American Journal of Hypertension* 13 (2000): 1250–55.

14. From Baroreceptors to Free Radicals

Carlson, J. T., et al. "Augmented resting sympathetic activity in awake patients with obstructive sleep apnea." *Chest* 103 (1993): 1763–68.

Dyugovskaya, L., P. Lavie, and L. Lavie. "Increased adhesion molecules expression and production of reactive oxygen species in leukocytes of sleep apnea patients." *American Journal of Respiratory and Critical Care Medicine* 165 (2002): 934–39.

Ip, M. S., et al. "Circulating nitric oxide is suppressed in obstructive sleep apnea and is reversed by nasal continuous positive airway pressure." *American Journal of Respiratory and Critical Care Medicine* 162 (2000): 2166–71.

Lavie, L. "Obstructive sleep apnoea—An oxidative stress disorder." *Sleep Medicine Reviews* 7 (2003): 35–51.

Ross, R. "Cell biology of atherosclerosis." *Annual Review of Physiology* 57 (1995): 791–804.

Somers, V. K., et al. "Sympathetic neural mechanisms in obstructive sleep apnea." *Journal of Clinical Investigation* 96 (1995): 1897–1904.

15. Death at an Early Age and the Paradox of Old Age

He, J., et al. "Mortality and apnea index in obstructive sleep apnea, experience in 385 male patients." *Chest* 94 (1988): 9–14.

Lavie, L. "Plasma vascular endothelial growth factor (VEGF) in sleep apnea syndrome: Effects of CPAP treatment." *American Journal of Respiratory and Critical Care Medicine* 165 (2002): 1624–28.

Lavie, P., et al. "Mortality in sleep apnea patients, a multivariate analysis of risk factors." *Sleep* 18 (1995): 149–57.

Lindberg, E., et al. "Increased mortality among sleepy snorers: A prospective population-based study." *Thorax* 53 (1998): 631–37.

Veale, D., et al. "Mortality of sleep apnoea patients treated by nasal continuous positive airway pressure registered in the ANTADIR observatory, Association Nationale pour le Traitement a Domicile de l'insuffisance respiratoire chronique." *European Respiratory Journal* 15 (2000): 326–31.

16. Treatments for Sleep Apnea Syndrome

Barvaux, V. A., G. Aubert, and D. O. Rodenstein. "Weight loss as a treatment for obstructive sleep apnoea." *Sleep Medicine Reviews* 4 (2000): 435–52.

Bettega, G., et al. "Obstructive sleep apnea syndrome, fifty-one consecutive patients treated by maxillofacial surgery." *American Journal of Respiratory and Critical Care Medicine* 162 (2000): 641–49.

Cartwright, R. "What's new in oral appliances for snoring and sleep apnea: An update." *Sleep Medicine Reviews* 5 (2001): 25–32.

Charuzi, I., et al. "Bariatric surgery in morbidly obese sleep-apnea patients: Short and long-term follow-up." *American Journal of Clinical Nutrition* 55 (1992): 594S-96S.

Clark, G. T., et al. "A crossover study comparing the efficacy of continuous positive airway pressure with anterior mandibular positioning devices on patients with obstructive sleep apnea." *Chest* 109 (1996): 1477–83.

Coccagna, G., et al. "Tracheostomy in hypersomnia with periodic breathing." *Bulletin of Physiopathologic Respiration* (Bulletin de Physiopathologie Respiratoire) 8 (1972): 1217–27.

Hudgel, D. W., and S. Thanakitcharus. "Pharmacologic treatment of sleep-disordered breathing." *American Journal of Respiratory and Critical Care Medicine* 158 (1998): 691–99.

Nathan, H., et al. "Mutilation of the uvula among Bedouins of the South Sinai." *Israel Journal of Medical Sciences* 18 (1982): 774–78.

Oksenberg, A., et al. "Positional vs. nonpositional obstructive sleep apnea patients: Anthropomorphic, nocturnal polysomnographic, and multiple sleep latency test data." *Chest* 112 (1997): 629–39.

Powell, N. B., R. W. Riley, and A. Robinson. "Surgical management of obstructive sleep apnea syndrome." *Clinics in Chest Medicine* 19 (1998): 77–86.

Schwartz, A. R., et al. "Therapeutic electrical stimulation of the hypoglossal nerve in obstructive sleep apnea." *Archives of Otolaryngology and Head and Neck Surgery* 127 (2001): 1216–23.

17. Sleeping Under Pressure—The Big Promise

Berry, R. B. "Improving CPAP compliance—man more than machine." *Sleep Medicine* 1 (2000): 175–78.

Findley, L., et al. "Treatment with nasal CPAP decreases automobile accidents in patients with sleep apnea." *American Journal of Respiratory and Critical Care Medicine* 161 (2000): 857–59.

Hack, M., et al. "Randomised prospective parallel trial of a therapeutic versus subtherapeutic nasal continuous positive airway pressure on simulated steering performance in patients with obstructive sleep apnoea." *Thorax* 55 (2000): 224–31.

Hedner, J., et al. "Reduction in sympathetic activity after long-term CPAP treatment in sleep apnoea: Cardiovascular implications." *European Respiratory Journal* 8 (1995): 222–29.

Jenkinson, C., et al. "Long-term benefits in self-reported health status of nasal continuous positive airway pressure therapy for obstructive sleep apnoea." *Quarterly Journal of Medicine* 94 (2001): 95–99.

Sullivan, C. E., et al. "Reversal of obstructive sleep apnoea by continuous positive airway pressure applied through the nares." *Lancet* 1 (1981): 862–65.

Wright, J., et al. "The health effects of obstructive sleep apnea and the effectiveness of continuous positive airways pressure: A systematic review of the evidence." *British Medical Journal* 314 (1997): 851–60.

18. A Whole New Understanding

Ball, E. M., et al. "Diagnosis and treatment of sleep apnea within the community, the Walla Walla project." *Archives of Internal Medicine* 157 (1997): 419–24.

Dement, W. C., and M. M. Mitler. "It's time to wake up to the importance of sleep disorders." *Journal of the American Medical Association* 269 (1993): 1548–50.

Kramer, N. R., et al. "The role of the primary care physician in recognizing obstructive sleep apnea." *Archives of Internal Medicine* 159 (1999): 965–68.

Lavie, P. "Physician education in sleep disorders—a dean of medicine's viewpoint." *Sleep* 16 (1993): 760–61.

Index

Illustrations are indicated in italic type

upper airways (continued)
treating blockages (*see* treatment for
sleep breathing disorders)
upper airway resistance syndrome,
76–78
See also nasal breathing
UPPP (uvulopalatopharyngeal plastic
surgery), 201–3
uvula, 95, *96,* 97, 201–3
uvulopalatopharyngeal plastic surgery
(UPPP), 201–3

vacuum pump, 5–6, 7
vagus nerve, 13, 65
vascular endothelial growth factor
(VEGF), 193–94
veins, 8. *See also* circulatory system
Virginia, 94

wakefulness
levels, 130 (*see also* daytime sleepiness, excessive)
mechanism, 69–70, 188 (*see also*
awakenings, nocturnal)
and voluntary vs. automatic respiratory control, 16–17
Walla Walla, Wash., 234–35
Webb, Bernie, 54
Wehr, Tom, 150
weight. *See* obesity; weight loss
weightlessness, effects of on sleep,
75–76, 119, 209
weight loss
after pharyngeal surgery, 202–3
apnea frequency reduced after, 92,
195
difficulty of, 50, 195, 196, 199

improvement in symptoms after, 24,
41, 43, 47, 50, 196–99
methods, 195–97
See also obesity
Weitzman, Elliot, 63, 70–72
Wells, W. D., 31–32
White, David, 74–75, 107, 225. *See
also* Harvard University School of
Medicine
white blood cells, 186, 230. *See also*
adhesive molecules
Wisconsin, University of, sleep research
at, 86–89. *See also* Wisconsin civil
servants study
Wisconsin civil servants study, 86–89,
92, 108, 127, 174, 227
women
complaints different than men's, 108
insomnia in, 83
partners of snorers/sleep apnea
patients, 105, 115, 121, 123
Pickwickian patients, 43–44, 104–5
prevalence of sleep apnea syndrome,
62–63, 85, 88, 106, 109
response to airflow resistance, 107
(*see also* upper airways)
seen less often in sleep laboratories,
107–8
sex hormones and sleep apnea, 106–7
(*see also* sex hormones)
sleep apnea mortality rates, 192
snoring, 80–81, 82, 98, 99, 108
See also gender
Wright, John, 169

Yanagisawa, Masashi, 141–42
Young, Terry, 87–89, 174, 227. *See also*
Wisconsin civil servants study